The Cure is in the Living

MY JOURNEY WITH CANCER

b

COLLEGE BOY
PUBLISHING

"We Breed Bestsellers"

Spirituality/Christian/Self-Help/Biographies

ISBN: 978-1-944110-49-9

Edited by **Armani Valentino & LaTangela Vann**
for College Boy Publishing
Published for Print and Digital formats by **Armani Valentino** for
College Boy Publishing
Cover Design by **Armani Valentino**
for College Boy Publishing

Published in Dallas, TX, by College Boy Publishing. College Boy Publishing is a division of The College Boy Company & ArmaniValentino.com. To order wholesale or bulk orders of this book, please contact the publisher directly at collegeboypublishing@gmail.com or call 972-383-9324.

Autographed copies of this book may be ordered directly from www.TheCureIsInTheLiving.com

Please allow up to 7-14 Business Days for delivery.

Barbara Downie is available for keynote addresses, workshops, panel discussions, consultations, and radio & television interviews by emailing thecureisintheliving@gmail.com or by calling 352-875-6300

Scriptures used come from the following:

New International Version (NIV) © Zondervon. All rights reserved.

Good News Bible (GNB) Good News Translation® (Today's English Version, Second Edition) Copyright © 1992 American Bible Society. All rights reserved.

King James Version

Printed in the United States of America
08 09 10 11 12 BDAV 5 4 3 2 1

The Cure is in the Living

MY JOURNEY WITH CANCER

Written by

BARBARA DOWNIE

In memory of my youngest brother,

the late **Dwight Downie**.

The Cure Is In The Living

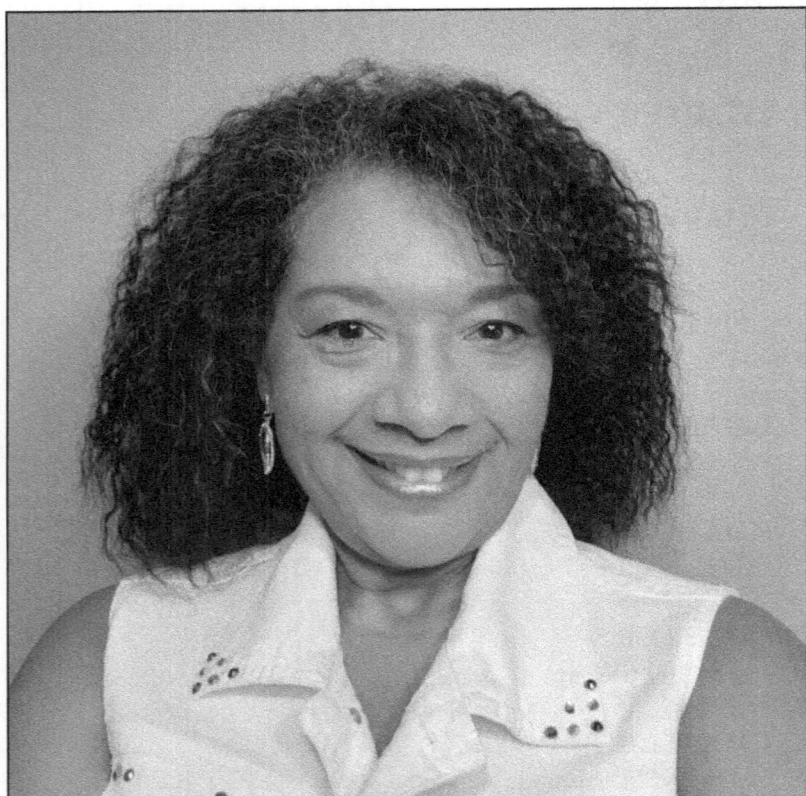

Introduction

    My first literary piece was a poem to my best friend while living in Jamaica, a gift for her sixteenth birthday. Her disbelief that I could have written such a nice poem encouraged me to put my thoughts in writing for decades to follow. I never shared most of my writings with the public, but my desire to write never died. That intense desire to share my experiences came as cancer threatened my life the second time. My multiple bouts with the disease heightened my experience with God's goodness, possible cures, disappointments, and overall spiritual growth with my Lord and Savior.

    Originally, the writing of this book began when cancer started to affect my life. However, I was persuaded to share more about my life growing up in Jamaica, West Indies. This suggestion delayed the book for another four months, because I feared sharing my experiences might be misunderstood and not be received well. After constant prayer, the words that guided me were "get out of the way." Realizing that the purpose of the book was to share my experiences with the hope of encouraging others and not what others think of me, I was able to share the good and the not-so-pleasant. parts

    This book is in no way providing medical advice or cures but simply sharing my experiences as I navigated through the pains and joys of my life and the source of my endurance.

    I pray that you are able to benefit and find that the cure is truly in the living and appreciating this thing we call life.

Peace and Blessings!

Barbara

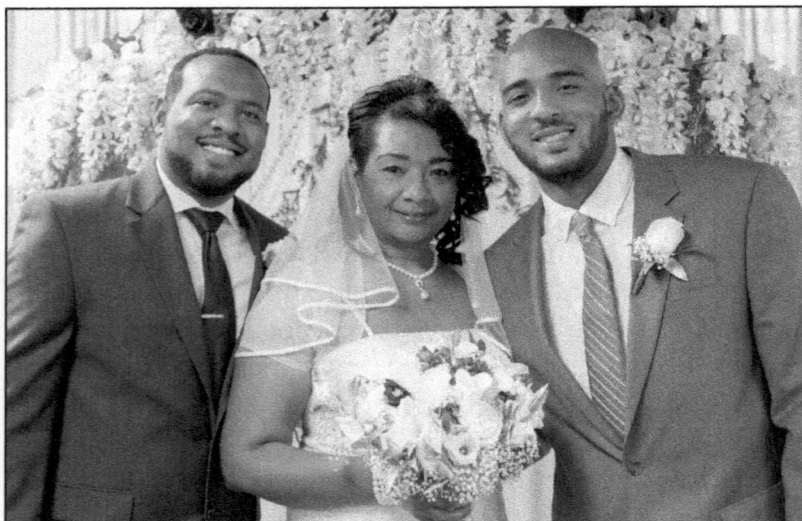

Mikey, Barbara, Nathan
(L-R)

"Trust in the Lord with all your heart.
Never rely on what you think you know.
Remember the Lord in everything you do,
and He will show you the right way."
Proverbs 3:5-6 (GNB)

Dedication

This book is dedicated to my sons Michael Morris, Jr. and Nathan Morris. You continue to be my biggest supporters and my hardest critics. I love you both more than words can ever tell. Thank you for the laughter over the years and for fathering my granddaughters, Mya and Olivia. Oh, how blessed I am to be their grandmother.

Thanks to my husband, Roger Thomas, for giving me all the support, time, and space I needed to complete this book.

A special thanks to all those who supported my endeavor, especially LaShaunn Elkins, the first person to read my first draft, and her encouragement to complete it.

Chapter 1

From the Past

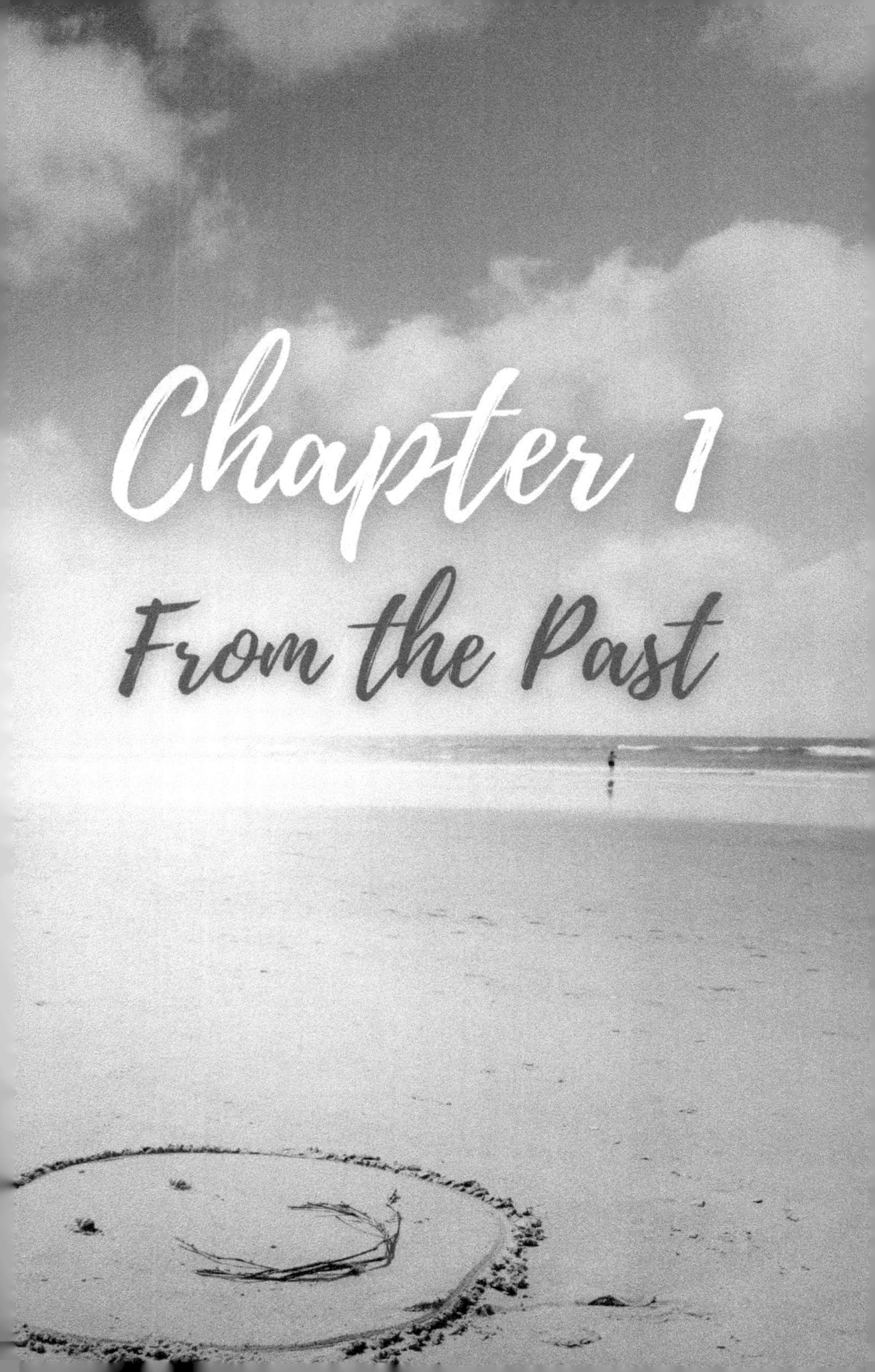

It was around the year 1985, and I was working as a Secretary in the Nutritional Services department of a major hospital in Ft. Lauderdale, Florida. It was lunch break, and I had just joined my friends in the cafeteria's dining room. As I occupied the last available chair around the table, the others were already engulfed in a conversation about a product and whether it worked or not. My only contribution to the discussion was, "Things never seem to work for me, even when others claim that it works great. In fact, with my luck, I would be one of those people who get cancer." As quickly as those words were spoken, they were forgotten.

More often than not, the early part of our lives usually shapes our future character and influences our thinking. My experiences growing up in **Jamaica** may raise a few eyebrows or cause a few gasps. Regardless of my own experiences, we all encounter different traumas. For some, it was sexual, physical, and or mental abuse. For others, it was abandonment, poverty, and mental handicaps. We can add so many different circumstances that have contributed to us being the people we are today.

During an interview, I heard an actor say that he knew he was destined to be famous from a very young age, and just as he said it, I could relate to what he was saying. I did not think I would be famous, but I, too, from a very young age, knew I was unique to God. It was not a prideful thing. In fact, the time I felt it, I did not understand why or even what to do with it, but it came alive when I heard the actor's words.

A turn in my journey of experiencing God's presence in my life began the afternoon of May 13, 1962, when my birth mother Clair started her 13 day trip by ship to London, England. She later described that day as being overwhelmed with mixed feelings. On the one hand, the possibility of making a better life was before her, and on the other hand, she had to leave her children behind to obtain it. She had made a choice and held on to the lifeline that became available, hoping to have her children join her later.

My father orchestrated my new guardians by asking Aunt Dine and Uncle Vincent to care for me in my mother's absence. He had also given her a clear warning not to forget me. Yet, at the innocent age of two years and five months old, the stigma of abandonment and inferiority was already attached to my life.

By age six, Claire had left and my time with Aunt Dine had ended. I was living with my father and his wife Judith in Springfield, St. Thomas, an eastern Parish in the Caribbean Island of Jamaica. I was now a part of a family unit, and had a new mother figure that would be the only mother I would know for years to come.

The view from the front of the two-bedroom rented property where we lived was a large sugarcane field. The distance between the two was an average-sized two-lane asphalted road with a gravel walkway on both sides of the street. There was a spot large enough to park two cars that extended beyond the first row of the vegetation. If my grandfather intended to visit for more than a few minutes, he would park his car across the street in that spot. On one of those visits, he took me across the street to his car, and I was able to finally touch what I had admired from across the street. Up close, it was like a wall of large, tall blades of grass swaying in the wind, extending way over my four (4) foot frame.

I can still remember a Sunday afternoon; some of my mother's friends came over to see my baby sister, the new arrival and addition to the family. I was dressed and told to sit on the veranda while the grown folks visited. Like most

Chapter One—From the Past

youngsters my age, I sat there playing by myself when I heard someone say, "do you know that God loves you?" I looked up to see a white-skinned man dressed in a yellow shirt and brown pants standing by the left post of the wrought iron front gate. In fear, I looked to the front door to see if an adult was standing there – I saw no one. I looked back at the gate, and the man was gone. As far as I could see up, down, and across the street to the cane field, there was no one in sight.

You might ask what is so strange about this. Well, St. Thomas is what we call 'the country.' We do not have tourists walking our streets, nor do we have any of them living there. It was the first time I had seen a Caucasian person, and he did not speak the way we do. In my dialect, the words would have been "yuh kno sey God love yuh?' with the word 'pickney' possibly added at the beginning or end of the question.

I did not tell anyone fearing they would not believe me, but I knew what I saw and heard. Although I did not know what it meant at the time, over the years, I have never forgotten the experience; it was forever etched in my mind, and always remembered the man's words, "Do you know that God loves you?"

Growing up, I went to both public and private schools. Religion was part of my life during my pre-teen years when I was a student of Holy Rosary proprietary school. As its name implies, it was a Catholic school. I attended mass, which was required for all students, and learned the Hail Mary, Glory Be, the Apostle's Creed, and The Lord's Prayer. These sayings were among others that I recited in responsive prayer. I obediently walked with the Nuns, dressed in full Habits, along with students as they paraded around the school and church carrying a replica representing the Virgin Mary crowned and adorned with flowers.

All the prayers and acts had no significant meaning to me. I knew I was not Catholic – nor did they try to convert me. I participated in their rituals because when it was devotion or special celebration times, all were expected to follow along. I was exposed to and learned about a culture I probably would not have known unless I attended this school. It was at this same school I found out that I had a hidden temper.

My classroom was one of several connecting rooms located at the far end of the property. These rows of classrooms were parallel to the back security wall, which separated the school from the surrounding businesses and homes in the neighborhood. The main doors led to the courtyard, and a back door opened up to a passageway between the building and that wall. One day as I exited the back door, a boy who was always teasing me was standing against the wall, and as he saw me, he started his usual verbal attack. While I have no recollection of what he did, I can never seem to forget that it made me angry enough that I walked up to him, clenched my fist, closed my eyes, and swung at him. The pain I felt and blood on my knuckles was not from my contact with the boy's face but instead from me hitting the rough unpaved concrete wall when the boy ducked to avoid my hand. Lesson learned; keep your eyes on the target.

I was sensible enough to notice how angry I felt and the trouble I would have been in if my hands met his face instead of the cement wall.

The second time I displayed such anger was one morning as I was getting ready for school at the home where I was boarding. I attended a private school away from home,

Chapter One—From the Past

so I lived with a family friend. Two of the girls there had the day off from their school and teased me about the fact that I had to go to school, and they did not. They took my uniform and tossed it back and forth to one another and would not allow me to get ready for school. As I pounced on the one holding the outfit, I did it again. I grabbed my uniform, closed my eyes, and swung my clenched fist at her. This time my fist made contact with the side of her forehead. She was light-skinned, so it took no time to show a red spot where my fist landed. I was horrified not because of what I did, but the trouble I thought I was in for hitting her. I knew I was going to be in trouble several times over – with her mother, my guardian, and my parents.

As if nothing had transpired, I put on my skirt and left for school before anyone started to ask questions. I figured the punishment would be awaiting me upon my return home, but when I got there, no one said anything, and I did not question why.

I was in a religious school, but none of it caused an early relationship with Christ. Back then, I did not thank God for keeping me from getting suspended from school or flogged for hitting someone. After all, I lived in a country and time when there was no age limit on getting flogged when you are under your parent's roof – or the equivalent of such. Is it possible that God saved me from the consequences of my actions even back then?

Those two incidents that could have caused a sore butt and back due to lashes from a belt, a switch from a tree, the garden hose, or any nearby object had revealed something to me about myself. I realized that if pushed, I can get angry enough to harm without thinking about the conse-quences –at the time. From that point, I made a conscious decision not to get into any confrontation with anyone. I got away with it twice; I might not the third time. Lesson learned, keep your emotions suppressed; a lesson that would cause damage to my future self.

This realization chartered my first step into becoming a passive individual. It became a big inner struggle as I avoided reacting to the action of others. People of authority who act first and listen later or behave in a superior manner that power gives them the go-ahead to mistreat and railroad others scare me. This experience proved to have a negative impression on my life for years to come.

Chapter 2

Money Is Not Automatic Happiness

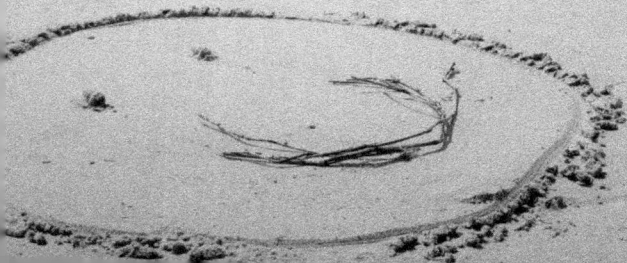

My understanding of God started in my High School years as I studied Religion and became more active in church, especially the youth group. This, however, did not minimize my constant feeling of inferiority. I was despised not only because of who my father was in stature but also for his roaming eyes and high consumption of alcohol. Nevertheless, neither vice kept him from his main passion, earning money – and he knew how to work for it.

I was disliked by many people because of the Downie name and the fact that I was the 'dead stamp' or the spitting image of my father. The size of my family in St. Thomas, Jamaica, was such that if a stranger simply mentioned the name Downie, it would most likely follow with the question "which one?"

Very few people did not know to which branch of the Downie family I belonged. Because of this, if I behaved unseemly on the route from school to the main town where we would walk to get public transportation, my mother would hear about it before I got home. Such transparency added another level to my passive behavior. I did not want to get in trouble, so I learned how to please others by being careful of my actions in public. I became a people pleaser, especially to those who could change the course of my life.

My life in High School was fun. I knew the group I would best fit in with, and it was not the popular group as I was not good enough for them. Having rich parents did not make you popular in our school; it was your intellect that made you popular and I was an average student. On the other hand, those I gravitated towards also thought I did not quite fit because my father had money. But they tolerated me anyway.

Using our society's scale to measure wealth within our community, most of my friends would not have moved the scale much. Yet, they were the wealthiest friends I had because they knew how to live and laugh regardless of their family's material possessions. There were always a few who would push the envelope, especially during lunch breaks. They didn't go around pretending to be better than others. They knew how to enjoy life and have fun, even if it meant getting in a little trouble sometimes.

We had our particular spot at the far end of the playing field, surrounded by trees and downslopes. A few of us would sit on large rocks at the top of the hill, laughing our heads off while being entertained by the daredevils of the group. They would slide down the narrow hill on coconut branches from the nearby trees. Call me chicken for not being adventurous, but I did not want to get my uniform soiled or explain to anyone why I was in such a state.

It was at one of these lunch periods when I learned that laughing while eating is not the right combination. On that unfortunate day, while sitting on my rock eating lunch, something caused me to start laughing suddenly, and before I could even figure what was happening, the food which should be going down my throat was painfully exiting my nose. Embarrassed and knowing I would become the next subject to be laughed at, I got up and set off for the restroom before anyone realized what had happened. The pain and discomfort continued for hours, but no one was the wiser of my mishap.

I can still visualize myself sitting on that big rock, dressed in my uniform; green jumper, white blouse, white socks, and black shoes. A few of my teachers often asked how I kept my socks so white and my black shoes so shiny and clean. I felt proud of my achievement and meant to keep it that way, and so every evening, I kept my appointment with a can of shoe polish and a soft brush.

Chapter Two
Money Is Not Automatic Happiness

In the classroom, I was an average student, but being liked was very important, as well as winning the hearts of some of the popular teachers. I knew the boundaries and tried not to cross them, but was also devious enough to know how to hide if I intended to go to the dark side. Well, maybe not entirely dark, how about the gray side?

I had learned many times from my siblings' mistakes. They had the habit of letting their guard down and spilling their heart out to our mother when they sat around talking and having a good time. But I knew better, because true to form of a Caribbean parent, when things are not so friendly, you will pay for the bad you did way back when. So I learned to listen and keep my secrets to myself. In a derogatory way, my mother would occasionally refer to me as 'Ms. Perfect'. Nothing could be further from the truth; I was just good at hiding my actions and feelings from those of authority – those who could hurt me if given a chance.

My angry person raised her ugly head one afternoon when a classmate who had never hidden the fact that she did not like me just would not let up. She thought I was rich and entitled and did not belong with the group of girls we hung out with. I did not want to be looked at as rich and defended my position to no avail. She kept laughing at everything I said and taunting me. Whatever I said to her was hateful enough to find myself outside the Principal's office, as directed by Mrs. Parker, the Principal's wife, who happened to be the teacher who entered the classroom right after the incident.

A result of having to go to the Principal's office, even in High School, meant being whipped in the palm of your hand with a very thin bamboo cane and your parents hearing about it as well. Luckily for me, the Principal was away that afternoon. After an hour of waiting, Mrs. Parker came by and was puzzled that I was still standing outside the office door. She took it upon herself to finally speak to me about the incident. When she found out that the other girl was the instigator, she verbally scolded me for my part and had me promise not to do it again, and sent me back to class. Needless to say, Rose was not happy, but I sure was. I feared my parents finding out more than the lashing from the cane. So I wonder again, did God keep me from the consequences of my actions? I did not close my eyes and swing this time, but my tongue sure cut deep that afternoon.

Outside of having to deal with the inferiority issues, school was where I laughed the most. At home, it was another matter. As much as I would like to share real times in this section of my life, I found it challenging to do so because when the good times came, more often than not, something negative came along and canceled it out. It's like always waiting for that other shoe to drop.

I didn't know what Clair, my birth mother looked like until age 15. That would be 12 years after she had left the island by ship to London, England, to make something of herself. I received letters and gifts over the years, but my emotional feeling towards her was nowhere near gratitude or thankfulness. I convinced myself that I disliked her and was afraid of feeling anything else. I felt that if I did not hate her, then I would hurt the feelings of those who had replaced her years of absence. I remember being deliberate with how I addressed her. The word mommy (as most Caribbean children address their mother) had never parted my lips in reference to her. I did not want to offend anyone.

It did not matter if my evaluation was right or wrong at the time, but that way of thinking caused more resentment

Chapter Two
Money Is Not Automatic Happiness

and fear to an already wounded and rejected soul. I quickly surmised that if I claimed that I did not like her, if I showed her faults, I would not be looked upon as ungrateful for my current situation. I know I am not alone. Can you remember saying you dislike someone because you knew you would be rejected by others if you did not? Well, that's the concept I had.

DISAPPOINTMENTS

Reaching the age of 16 is an exciting time for a teen-age girl, and I was no different. I had asked, and my mother agreed that I could have a sweet 16 birthday party. I invited all my friends; it was not many, but I was going to have a good time to remember.

A week before the party was to happen, my father came home, ate his dinner, and was heading for the bedroom when he asked me to wake him up at a specific time. However, that very same evening, I was already given the green light to go to an event at school. The time he needed me to wake him up was an hour after I needed to leave the house - and I did not want to miss this event. After all, school events were the only events I was allowed to attend on my own. Fearing him telling me to miss the event so I could wake him up, I did not say anything about my plans. After all, it was early evening, and he was already intoxicated and was about to fall asleep. With great anticipation of a wonderful evening, I went to my event.

I had a good time at school that evening. I loved drama, and the drama department was performing. The beauty of our school's layout was such that the classrooms, cafeteria, library and some offices created an elongated rectangle shaped border for the courtyard. When you enter from the main entrance and walk up to the school, at the far end of that four tiered courtyard was our stage with ample space for chairs as needed for viewers whenever we had an event. It was so strategically placed that anywhere you were standing, you would be able to see the performance on stage.

Viewing points were not limited to the courtyard. Sometimes we would stand by the railings outside the classrooms on the first floor or even from the hallways of the second and third floor. No matter where you stood, you could still see the stage in the courtyard. We had an outdoor theater and were often entertained under the stars. It also gave us giddy youngsters the ability to move about the grounds and still see the goings-on on stage, which also contributed to the fulfilled evening with my friends. I will be lying if I say that was the only exciting thing I did. We also knew about all the dark spots where the seniors hung out – necking. It was still during the days when keeping your virtue meant something, so any girl we saw in a dark place with a boy made for good gossip. For an almost sixteen-year-old girl, necking was something to look forward to, if anyone was bold enough to be my boyfriend.

The following day I learned how angry my father was. He did not scream or verbally scold me – he never did. He just decided he would not support me having a birthday party. In fear of him showing up drunk and humiliating me, my mother and I decided to cancel my sweet sixteen birthday party. The opportunity to celebrate a coming of age, a milestone in my life was lost, never to be regained.

If asked what the play was about and the number of couples we ran upon in the dark stairways, and the things we giggled about like immature teenage girls, I cannot recall.

Chapter Two
Money Is Not Automatic Happiness

But I never forgot the shame of having to tell everyone that my sweet sixteen birthday party was canceled.

At the end of each school year, we would have award ceremonies where the student with the highest points in a given subject within their grade-level would get an award. My favorite subject was Arts and Crafts, and I was above average in this area of studies. I did so well one year that my grades had me in first place for that subject.

A few of us had some specific projects we were working on for an upcoming art fair, and were allowed to complete our projects while the remaining class continued with the still object drawing session. Mrs. Brown told us she would keep the drawing display up so that those working on projects for the art fair could come in whenever we had free sessions to complete our drawings.

The following afternoon, I worked on the drawing assignment until it was time to go home. I finished my drawing and said goodbye to my teacher, who was sitting in her office in another room. When I returned the following day, my teacher asked me why I left the objects out instead of breaking them down and putting them away. I had no idea that was expected of me since the set-up was not created just for me, and I had no idea who was or was not coming after me to complete their project. Needless to say, that misunderstanding cost me the first place Arts and Craft subject award. My teacher did not give me the benefit of the doubt, and since she had to put the display away, she reduced my grade on that assignment. When I voiced my disagreement that what she was doing was unfair, her response was one which I will never forget; "All is fair in love and war."

Although I did not change her mind then, I still hoped that on awards day, I would hear my name called for that first place. Once again, all the hard work, the beautiful projects I designed and completed, and the pride of being recognized and acknowledged for being the best in something were lost.

For years, I witnessed the beauty of seniors walking across the stage in their cap and gown to accept their diplomas, and I anxiously waited for my turn. However, in the summer of 1977, when it came time for my graduation, our graduation team decided they did not want to wear graduation gowns; we had a few "want to be" Rastafarians in that year's graduation class. And so I was not able to walk across the stage in my cap and gown.

We also had more than enough space at the school to have the graduation dance, but no...they chose a dance hall (equivalent to a nightclub), so I did not attend my graduation dance either because my parents did not approve of the venue. Once again, I got there and it changed. I was once again left disappointed.

My sister, Deann, who calls herself the rebel, decided she was going to sneak out to go to a party with one of her girlfriends. My sister, who did not have a source of income, borrowed whatever money she needed from her friend for the party. They were both in their teens at the time, and I was not aware of her plans.

My sister got caught. When questioned where she got the money – thinking nothing of it, she stated that I gave it to her. She warned me after the fact, which made me upset, pointing out that she knows I am now going to be in trouble for something I did not do. I was walking up the stairs just in time to overhear a conversation between my parents. It was being surmised that Deann's confession was forced to protect me from my supposed indiscretion. Her attempt to set the record straight failed, and the blame still rests on me.

Chapter Two
Money Is Not Automatic Happiness

I asked myself, "What is wrong with me that others, without question, would believe the worst about me?" No one knew I overheard, and even though they saw me as the one at fault, I never corrected them. My passive behavior had reached maturity.

Someone once said that negative attention is better than no attention at all, but I feared negative attention; it is downright painful. So without realizing it, I would work hard to gain others' approval by not rocking the boat. With that, I learned not to get excited about things because, by the time I got to that point, things changed. After enough disappointments, my excuse for not trying started with the words, 'with my luck...'

DREAM

Date: November 6, 1980
Scene: Parent's house in Jamaica

It was my wedding day, but I was cleaning the house instead of getting myself ready for the wedding. It was getting late, and I ran upstairs to find a dress to change into when I saw the guy I was getting married to at the window, and he was upset because my clothes and hair were such a mess.

I grabbed a white dress from the closet (it was a dress that I owned) and tried it on to see if it would fit, but it was tight-fitting – I had gained weight.

I ran back downstairs, and as I was passing a lamp table, I saw the newspaper and picked it up. The date at the top of the newspaper read October 24, 1983. I WOKE UP with the realization that the date was three years in the future. I marked the date on a small 3x4 inch calendar and forgot about it.

The Cure Is In The Living

Chapter 3

Surviving on Fear

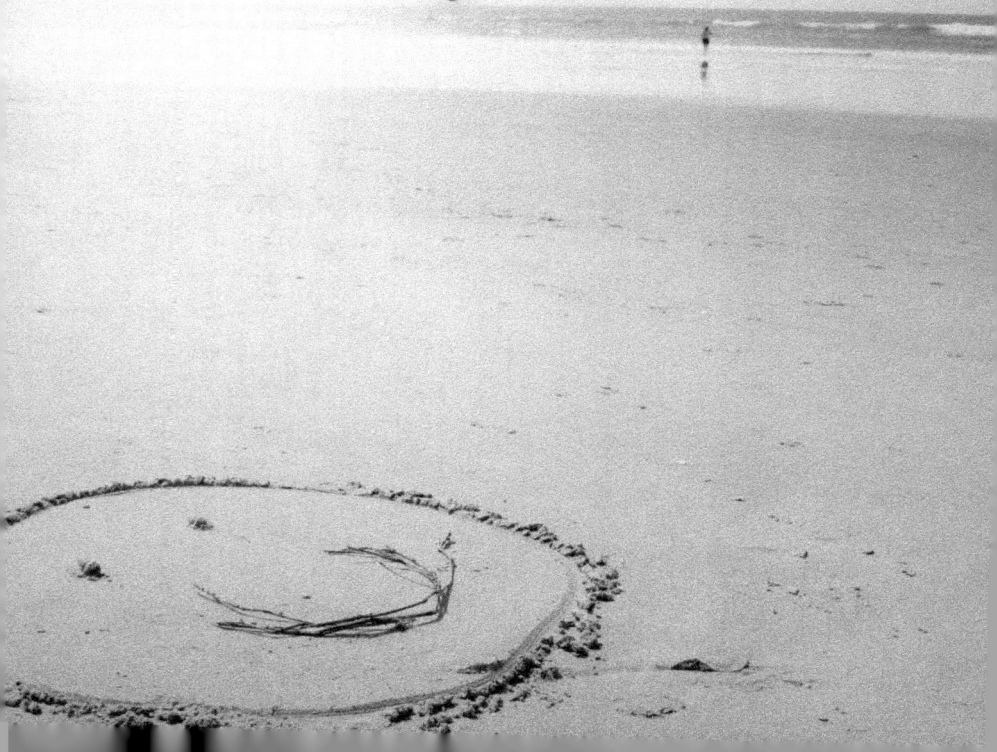

I moved to the United States in the winter of 1979, where I joined the Grey household as a guest until I fulfilled my father's plans to enroll in college. The idea was to major in Business Administration because it was my father's choice. Truth be told, I had no desires of my own, so I cannot say he forced me to do something I did not want to do. There were a lot of unknowns. Although I was weeks away from being 20 years old at the time, my life before was quite sheltered. What should have been a rather exciting time was more like another day in a new place - nothing to be excited about.

I was accustomed to doing as I was told and not to create a reason for anyone to be upset with me. I could still feel the possible ramifications of being shouted at or the feeling of inadequacy as if I was still home. My body was over five hundred and seventy miles away from Jamaica, but my mind never left home.

My earlier life experiences and environment shaped my personality. Even when freedom presented itself, at first, I continued to live a life of still trying to please my parents. It was as if they were always watching my every move.

With no experience under my belt, my first job was as a live-in maid. After a year of doing that and away from everyone who knew me or could report on my actions, I developed the confidence I needed to recognize and accept my freedom. I eventually got a part-time job at a hospital in Ft. Lauderdale, Florida. It worked for me at the time because I had to be a full-time student.

With school, work, and the realization that no authoritative eyes were watching over me, I received the advances of young men from school who showed interest – but I was different. I was not up on the latest fashions and styles, nor was I street smart (as they thought I should be). So no meaningful relationships were ever formed with my school-mates.

The Cure Is In The Living

I might have been somewhat sheltered, but I knew the type of guy that would interest me. I quickly found out that they preferred more popular girls who were socially outgoing and closet ready for the next weekend party. But, there was still hope for the non-social.

My parents owned a house in the United States, which was my home while I was in college. The person managing the house rented a section to a family friend's son and his wife. My daily routine didn't change much. The majority of the time, I went to school, the grocery store, and back home. And, in that order, perfectly mapped out on my bus route. There was a survival income from my dad with the underlying understanding that I needed to find a job, so it was not long after that I sought employment.

My parents did not know I did not have enough because I did not tell them when the hard times started. All due to my stubbornness and fear. You see, when I encountered my first winter in Florida, I was in the garage newly converted into a living space, so I found myself in need of a portable heater. My guardian relayed this deficiency to my father, and it came back to me that he had said I was old enough to get married and have someone take care of me. On that note, I was determined to make as much money as I could without asking for help. And that is what I did. It did not matter to me whether he meant it or not; I just knew that I did not want to give him the chance to repeat it, ever.

Food was scarce but I never felt that I was in a bad place, though. I knew my situation, and I faced it head-on; no complaints. Call it irony or divine appointment, but my hunger stage was about to diminish because I was now working in the Nutritional Services department at the hospital. Yep, there was a flicker of light at the end of the tunnel.

Chapter Three—Surviving On Fear

My first day on the job was observation only, but I took extensive notes, gathered sample diet kits and menus to take home with me. You would think I was preparing for an exam. Quite the contrary, remember, I am a people pleaser, and I planned to impress their socks off even if I was just working in the kitchen.

That night I familiarized myself with all the different types of menus and how they apply to patients. By my second day on the job, I knew what they were and how they were to be used and needed no one to show me how to set up the patient's trays to match their individual needs. By my third day, I was no longer in training but had a regular assignment. I learned the strategies of seasoned Diet Assistants and Aids on how to set up, serve, clean up, and clock out on time. It did not take long before I had proved myself and was trusted to handle an entire smaller floor by myself. I was dependable and asked to work on my days off or full shifts over the weekends when I did not have class.

Due to ongoing discharges and new patients coming in, the Diet Assistants would order a few extra entrees to compensate for a meal shortage situation. However, the rule was that staff members were not allowed to eat or take any unused food home but instead should dispose of it in the garbage at the end of the shift. I disobeyed that rule - somewhat. I was just not as bold as some to take home extra. Not because I did not think of it, but the benefit of having the food was way less to me than the embarrassment of being caught. However, being seen eating on the floor was way less embarrassing and much more comfortable for me to master. When I was hungry on the days I worked, and there was a leftover entrée that I liked, I ate. When there was none available, my favorite go-to would be Frosted Flakes cereal with banana and milk – depending on availability.

The lack was visible on my body. I had dropped from a size eight dress to a size one dress and was too silly to see it as unhealthy. Come on. I was 5 feet 8 inches tall wearing a size one dress. Who would not see some good in that? People are always trying to lose weight. But it did not last forever. The more hours I worked, the more I gained my weight back. Hmmm - I wonder why?

My only transportation was the bus with the closest stop at the entrance of the subdivision. At the other end of my route, there was another bus stop at the front of the college. When my father found out how difficult it was to walk from the house to the main street to get to the bus stop, especially during Florida's rainy season, he bought me a rust-colored hatchback Fiat car. I hated the color and its shape, but at least I had a car – sort of.

Two weeks into being a car owner and only driving to school and work, the tow truck had to take it to the mechanic. I was all ready for school one morning when I walked out with a book bag and keys in hand when I noticed a pinkish oil-like substance running down the driveway. Not being able to identify the problem, I called Mr. Pace, my dad's friend, told him the situation, and started my long walk to the bus stop.

On my way back from school, I got off at the stop close to Mr. Pace's office to see about the car to learn it was at the transmission shop. Luckily for my dad, he paid only for the initial repair even though it was back into the transmission shop within days of it being fixed. Thanks for the service warranty.

Something had to be done, but those in authority weren't saying anything. I surmise that if each repair were coming out of pocket, someone would be shouting. The next move had to be mine. I needed more money, so I made it known to those of influence at work that I was available for all possible overtime. My supervisors figured I was a fast learner, so there were no limits to where I could work. My job became full-time hours on weekends and my days off if needed, and it went back to part-time during the week.

By the end of nine months, it was time to drop my burden and ask Mr. Pace if he would cosign for a new car since I had no credit. He agreed, and I bought myself a base model Blue Toyota Corolla. It had no extras. It was a standard shift, did not have a radio, there were no stripes on the side (it was popular those days), but it was NEW and had air conditioning. So since I was the one who chose to buy a new car, I had no intention of complaining about my situation. Because of my low income, my father continued paying the car insurance on the new car as he intended to do with the Fiat. Thankfully, I did not have to pay rent. My pathway was getting brighter.

The Cure Is In The Living

Chapter 4

The Meeting

I met the man I would eventually be married to for 23 years right in my bedroom. No, it is not as steamy as you might be thinking, so let me explain. I didn't even own a television, so whenever my roommates were not using theirs, they would lend it to me. Although it was a three-bedroom house, we did not establish a common area and spent most of the time at home in our designated part of the house – the bedroom.

One evening after work, I was sitting in my room watching my borrowed black and white 11-inch screen TV when one of my housemates pushed his head around my door to tell me he wanted to introduce me to someone. I was appropriately dressed, and my bedroom door was open – so I said, "sure, bring him in," and so that is how I met Michael.

After our first meeting, we would glimpse each other and exchange a brief greeting occasionally when he came over to visit his friends. Every time I saw Michael, I noticed that he was always wearing a big knitted red, green, and gold cap, which caused me to think he was a Rastafarian covering his locks. Because of this, I had no interest in him beyond being casual friends. So imagine my surprise when he invited my mother and me to dinner when he learned she was coming to town. We have never even had a good conversation - and now dinner? With my mother? The person who has never approved of anyone who showed interest in me? Well, except for one guy, while I was still in Jamaica, but my father put a stop to that one. Word on the street was that he showed up at his house with a gun and told him to leave me alone – but I believe the gun element was a fabrication so that every young man in the district would leave Mr. Downie's daughter alone.

The Cure Is In The Living

Anyway, let's get back to Michael. Although I turned down the invitation, my mother thought it would be a good idea. So, dinner it was. It was the Friday night that ended my life as I knew it. You might be asking what changed, and you might also have guessed it, 'my mother liked him.'

My attitude towards Michael changed, not because I was necessarily interested, but because my mother approved of him.

I opened up and allowed Michael in my life – one that would no longer only consist of school, work, and home. I accepted his invitations, and we would go out and have a good time with other couples to movies or dinners on weekends. Still, I was not too fond of the party scenes. My closet did not house anything sexy enough to blend in, and my part-time job was barely paying for my car and food.

For the privilege to use a liquor store to cash his paycheck, Michael would purchase German, Italian or unusual wines. And so when he got paid, I got a bottle of wine. This experience was different – someone was paying attention to me, and I was having fun. The price of this lifestyle came at the expense of my studies. My grades started to drop, and I visited my counselor more often than I cared to do. However, I was experiencing life as I came to know it.

Our commitment was tested when my father came to the US on business and came by the house. Of course, while I knew how my mother felt, this did not determine how my father felt, so I asked Michael not to hang out at the house the way he had now become accustomed. Cut me some slack now; after all, my father was paying for my shelter and education.

I thought nothing of the request. In my mind, to deal with my father's disapproval versus my boyfriend being insulted was no comparison. It was only for a few days.

Chapter 4—The Meeting

It did not occur to me that something was or could even be wrong with my request until that night when I received a call from Michael's sister. Thinking that we had a falling out, she wanted to know what happened between us. I explained my side of the coin, and she gave me her opinion. I cannot remember what she said, but what stayed with me was that she cared about our relationship enough to make that call. Without her knowing it, her concern was another layer of approval for me. Seven months later, we were engaged.

There was a group of five of us, all Jamaicans, and we worked at the same hospital in Ft. Lauderdale. We were married at different times, but not too far apart from each other. I was last. They did the bridal shower ritual, which was a lot of fun. The practical person that I am, I still ask, "What is the use of lingerie that is uncomfortable to wear at any time and for any reason?" There were the usual smirks and 'oh yah' outburst as I opened each gift and held them up to show.

At that bridal shower were friendships and acquaintances developed over the past three years of me living an unrestricted life. It was to my great disappointment that none of these ladies would be able to travel to Jamaica for the wedding. Including Ann Marie, whom I had hoped to stand as my matron of honor; she had been the one who took me places and the catalyst to the relationships I now enjoyed.

The winter semester of 1983 was the semester for me to graduate. However, there was a conflict with scheduling. First, I desired to be a June bride, which would have worked perfectly; graduation from college in December and wedding the following June.

My mother, however, selected the month of December for the wedding. And 'as my luck' would have it, that year's finals were the same week of my pending wedding and honeymoon. Although I drew the line at getting married on the 10th, which was my birthday, I did not want to offend, so Dec 17th it was. You must be seeing a pattern by now to surmise already that I got married and did not do finals.

I landed in Jamaica the night of Thursday, Dec 15th, five days after my 24th birthday, and got married on Saturday, Dec 17th, following an 11-month engagement.

It was as if my wedding happened, and I was just there – as a guest. There was no great excitement of seeing my dream come to fruition. I had no control over it. The planning, the flowers, the cake, my bridesmaids; none of them were choices I made.

The type of flowers I wanted for the bouquets were not the ones I eventually had. I love to see baby's breaths in a wedding bouquet, and that is what I requested. Instead, in it were stems of feathery-like foliage, a very close resemblance to Asparagus Plumosus Fern. That filler in flower arrangements always reminded me of funerals because it was a constant in all funeral wreaths that I had seen, and I hated it. It was what I associated the foliage with that was the issue, not the appearance of it, so what's the big deal, right?

The simple three tier wedding cake I selected was replaced with eight cakes, four rounds and four squares, **and** in the middle was a 12 inch round cake topped with another 10 inch round. On top of those cakes was a plastic base and four six-inch roman columns to support the other two rounds, the 10-inch and 8-inch cakes. On both sides of the center tower, we had the 12 x 12 square cakes at the bottom, also supporting plastic bases and six-inch roman columns to

Chapter 4—The Meeting

hold the 8 x 8-inch square cakes.

To complete the presentation, they had the best feature of all; plastic staircases from the center tiers leading to the two side towers. The staircase on the left had three male figures, and on the right, there were three female figures. All figures were dressed in the same color scheme as the actual bridal party. And, of course, the bride and groom wedding topper was perched on the top of the center tier. It was quite the masterpiece.

Everyone involved in creating the event had put their all in it, many late nights and hard work. It was indeed a momentous occasion with the best Caribbean style foods fit for a wedding. But for me, it was not "my" wedding. My friends were in the United States. Therefore, my parent's friends made up the majority of the wedding guests, and rightly so, it was, after all, their event; they planned, paid, and executed. I kept quiet and compliant.

Being fearful is a crippling place to be. Let us examine the facts. I was a few credit hours away from graduation, so the threat of my parents not paying my tuition would not affect me much. I had already started planning my wedding in the United States on a much smaller scale. So, the threat of not getting my wedding paid for was no big deal. I would have had a wedding anyway. I still would have been a married woman. Also, the fear of being thrown out of my father's house was no longer an issue. The most significant issue and ultimately the saddest was not my mother wanting to give the most lavish wedding, but my fear of offending others and avoiding confrontation.

I went to Jamaica for a couple weeks, got married, enjoyed a honeymoon on the coast, and then returned to the United States. As soon as I got back, I jumped right back into the swing of things. The first order of business was to schedule a doctor's appointment, which confirmed what I suspected for the past two weeks. I was pregnant.

Apart from the expected morning sicknesses, I had a very healthy pregnancy and kept pace with work and home. I loved shopping for the baby, and I found my favorite baby store neatly tucked away on Commercial Boulevard. I was very independent and did not need anyone to accompany me when I went shopping. I would get in my car, and off I would go. I had all the time just to look and leave without buying anything. Compulsive, I am not.

It is customary for me to walk into a store, pick up something I like, and walk around the store looking at other items. All the while, I was evaluating if the thing I had in my hand was a need or want, and I would put it back if it did not prove to be absolutely necessary. Who would want someone breathing down their neck with a shopping habit like that?

Most definitely, I too had the first baby syndrome, and everything needed to be perfect – as possible for my limited means. I liked sewing, and I figured it would be great to make a comforter set for my baby, and so I did. I chose two different color cotton materials; yellow and white stripe and green and white stripe. My signature project was a baby comforter, diaper bag, and pillow sham. For the comforter, I used the green material for the back. The front had a checker pattern of both the green and yellow stripe material, with each alternate square embroidered with the shape of an animal or building blocks. I finished it off with a white eyelet frilled edge. The diaper bag had the top quarter made with the yellow material, and on the remainder of the bag, I used the green. The pillow was more straightforward, green on one side, yellow on the other, and surrounded with the white eyelet border. I was proud of my accomplishment as I stood

Chapter 4—The Meeting

back and looked at everything in place, adorning the baby's white furniture. I did it all – all except the embroidery, which was done by my mother-in-law at the time.

On July 24th, I had a healthy baby boy. He was named Michael Jr., but before long, we called him Mikey. He was delivered at the same hospital where I worked. There was an advantage to being an employee. I was in familiar surroundings since I had walked those halls many times over the past couple of years. The icing on the cake was the fact that I had the privilege of having one special meal. For one day, my dinner tray did not have a product derived from a frozen prepackaged meal, but instead, it was a small lobster tail, baked potato, green beans, and a garden salad on the side. And to satisfy my sweet tooth, my favorite, a slice of cheesecake with glazed cherry topping. No, I did not have a tiny vase with a flower though that would have been nice. Anyway, the takeaway here was not the fancy meal itself but because it made me feel important. And that was reiterated when my doctor came in for his afternoon visit, noticed my tray, and commented, "I did not know you were a celebrity around here." Little did he know, I felt like a nobody on the inside.

My husband and I did not attend church regularly, so we had to ride on my in-laws tails to have the baby christened at their church. While I never lost sight of who God is, I was not going to church, reading the scriptures, or praying much. However, something special happened after that Sunday when Mikey got baptized, because his father decided that we should start attending church regularly. And so we did. *It was a move that would change my life with Christ forever.*

By our first anniversary celebration, when my parents came to visit during the Christmas holiday, they were a little upset that we had a get together with friends at the house. After this, we decided to rent an apartment. I was 26 years old, and for the first time, I felt free from being under my parent's rule. Wow, how pathetic!

While unpacking from this move, I found that 3x4 calendar where I wrote the date October 24, 1983, from the dream I had November 6, 1980. It was now January 1985, and I realized that October was the month I got pregnant. My son's birth date is the 24th, and the year I got married was 1983. Wow, how exciting!

Chapter 5

When the Honeymoon is Over

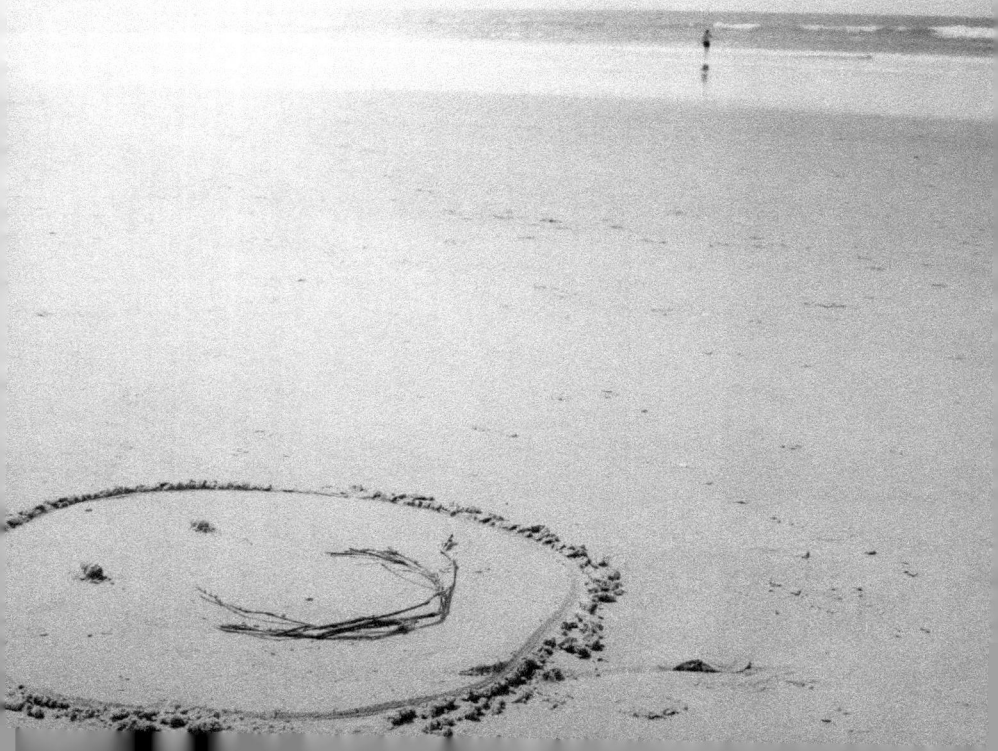

Things started to get shaky. It was my husband's birthday, a month shy of our 2nd wedding anniversary. He came home with 11 red roses. I inquired, where was the 12th? He just brushed it off, saying that the staff at his office had given him the flowers for his birthday and that someone came and pulled one out of it. I left it alone at that point. A couple of hours later, he said he would be back in a minute. However, he didn't return home until early the next morning, something he had never done before.

I asked what was going on? It was apparent that another woman was the reason he didn't come home. He remained quiet while I argued. Eventually, he told me not to worry about it, to leave it alone, and it won't happen again. I kept pushing for an explanation. It upset him at that point where he slapped me across the cheeks.

It is incredible how quickly things can go through your mind in the moments before reality occurs. I immediately remembered the ways of my father and how abusive he was, and my many declarations that I would not endure such treatment. Right now, I was smack dab in the middle of such a situation. As my head swung forward, so did my fisted right hand. I hit him back and stood there looking straight in his eyes. From his facial expression, I think he was shocked not only at my response but that he hit me. He hesitated, followed by a slight push, and told me to get away from him. At this juncture, something else also came over me, and that was fear of what I could be angered to do if I reached the point of closing my eyes. It also became apparent that it wasn't going in the direction that I wanted because he wasn't going to divulge any information. I felt I was the one to be blamed since I kept pursuing an answer for his actions. I walked away, but not before telling him he had no right to hit me. What I was thinking and what I said did not quite complement each other because I was scared – but I was not about to show it. No one must know my true feelings.

After that incident, there was no evidence of the affair or odd behavior, so I had no reason to question his actions. But I was being careful and decided not to have another child, being leery of what was going on with our relationship.

Things appeared to be normal for several years until I became pregnant with my 2nd child. I guess the mistress, who had been dormant, felt shafted when she found out from an acquaintance that the wife was pregnant. She somehow thought she had an obligation to make me aware of her existence and that she did by her telephone calls to our home.

The months that followed were full of arguments, much crying, and disbelief that the life I swore not to live, I was living. My son Nathan made his entrance into the world on March 10th, a few years after his brother. He was only a week old when my husband went out for the evening supposedly to hang with friends. I developed a fever during the evening and felt downright exhausted dealing with a newborn and a four-year-old. I put Mikey into bed early, but it was not so simple for an always crying newborn. Breastfeeding my children was my choice, but because of high-grade fever, I decided to switch to using formula until I got better.

At that time and with my Caribbean upbringing pouring formula in a bottle and sticking it in a microwave was not the option. Instead, the baby nipples and glass bottles had to be sterilized, and water boiled to be added to the powdered formula. The smell of the baby formula was such a reminiscence of the one I used to feed my baby brother when I was ten years old. I just loved the smell of it and chose powder over liquid formula.

Chapter 5—When the Honeymoon is Over

It was past one o'clock the following morning when my husband came home to find me fixing a bottle for the late -night feeding. Boy, did I have a lot to say about the situation. I was not the only one responsible for this child. It was unfair for him to be out so late, leaving me to deal with it all – not to mention that I was sick myself... Yep, I was very vocal as I handed him the bottle, insisting he should be the one to do that feeding so I can get some rest.

Amid my warranted complaining of how inconsiderate he was, he turned to get the baby from the crib, and I noticed something red on the back of his shirt collar. As I looked closer, I realized it was the tag on his shirt. The fact that his shirt was inside out meant he had taken that shirt off and put it back on after he left the house that evening. Angrily I revealed what I observed and accused him of being out with a woman. No matter what I said - he did not utter a word, which angered me even more. "Who knows where you have been?" I blurted in disgust as I took my child out of his hands and demanded that he leave the room.

All I could think was, *What am I going to do? I now have two children and my life is heading in the wrong direction.*

The Cure Is In The Living

Chapter 6

Keep On Running

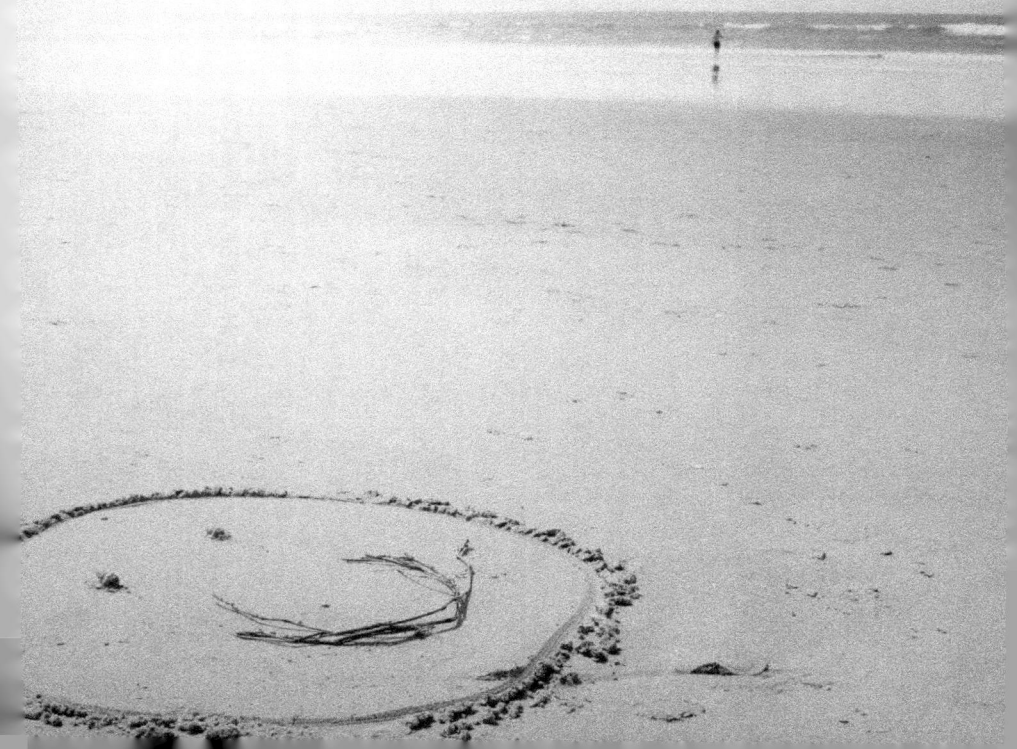

Outside of an auto accident that caused a herniated disk in my upper body, I had no health issues. But around June 1990, tests showed cancerous cells in my cervix, and a month afterward, I had a total Hysterectomy.

Following that major surgery, every year around June – July, I would be in pain from one thing or another. I had fluid on my knee, body aches, weakness, and a ruptured eardrum, but no matter the issues, the doctors could not identify the cause – all the tests they did were inconclusive to my condition. I would battle the constant pain and doctor's visits to the beginning of the following year, between February and March, when the ailment would simply stop. The attacks would repeat yearly, but it took several years before I realized the pattern.

Ft. Lauderdale was getting crowded. Many were relocating north from Dade county after tropical storm Andrew passed directly through the city of Homestead as a category five hurricane, causing massive destruction throughout parts of that County areas. We relocated further north as well to Ocala, FL, in 1996 with the notion that it would be a peaceful place to be and ultimately a better environment for our young boys.

I timed the move to fit their next level of education so that they would not have to do half term in Ft. Lauderdale and the other in Ocala. Mikey had just finished Elementary and was about to enter Middle School. I figured he had a good foundation to enter the public school system. Nathan, the pistol out of the two, was entering elementary and was registered to attend private school, just like his brother did at that age. The plan had been that our children started in Christian private schools through to their elementary years to create a Christian foundation for them. What I learned, though, is that the private schools can select or reject whomever they want to and did not have any obligation to spend time caring for a disobedient child. This low tolerance created a problem with Nathan, the pistol I mentioned earlier. He had only two years in that environment. His first-grade teacher related to him so well. At the end of that year, he received the "most improved student" award. But his second year was more challenging. His new teacher did not have the time to figure out how to get the best out of him. She was more concerned that he might be a bad influence on the other children but did not prove to be the case when things were reversed.

I remember Nathan telling me one evening that he was scared of one of the boys because he told Nathan that he was going to have his father shoot him. Mother bear went into action and scheduled a meeting with the teacher and the Principal because the teacher had done nothing when Nathan had complained. Imagine my surprise when I learned that she actually heard the threat but thought nothing of it. The Principal agreed with me that the teacher should have done more to assure my child that he was safe and went into his spiel that all children should feel safe, etc.

My mind had already started to plan a move; this was not worth all the money I was paying out each month. Plus, I did not trust that this incident would not cause negative repercussions against Nathan, nor did I want him to experience being expelled from this school. He was very observant and had already adopted a negative stigma from his ADHD diagnosis. I can recall how it took my breath away one morning when I heard him say, "I know I am stupid" he was only four years old, so someone had already planted that thought. It became my mission to reverse those thoughts.

Chapter 6—Keep On Running

Moving to Ocala was a shock in all phases. My first permanent job in Ocala was working at a garbage company. I was the secretary to two brothers in their family-owned company. I was a tad embarrassed to be working for a garbage company, but every other job I was sent to by Girl Friday employment agency thought I was overqualified. I tried to convince them that I would be loyal, pointing out my 15 years at my previous employment but without success. The garbage company, however, often told me that the ninth was the charm as they had interviewed eight people before me and did not like them.

These men were strong-willed, opinionated, yet kind, and overall good business people but not a group with whom you'd want to butt heads. Comply with their instructions, work hard, and acknowledge their authority, and you will be ok. I noticed most of all, how tightly knit this family was, and I was impressed by that. If I shared the fact that I worked for this family with anyone who has done business with them, they would always (cannot remember an exception) sympathize with me, but I could not relate to why they needed to. I was hired to do the work, and I strived to do it well. I learned who they wanted to speak with directly and those they wished to avoid for a while. At an event a man told one of the brothers that it's like dealing with Fort Knox to get past his secretary to talk to him.

One brother liked his visitors served beverages in glasses or real coffee cups; the other it was not all that important. I studied their differences and left no room for criticism or confrontation. I am the master people pleaser; I had learned to treat a person how they want to be treated. My relationship with the entire family was one that edged on the border of employee and employer. Still, I never lost sight of my actual position and that the blurred line was simply due to genuine kindness and respect for my work. In my opinion, I was a professional and professionalism, and being the best and having the best was the very essence of who these brothers were.

We parted ways when the company was sold, and it was hard to pack up and watch them leave. I no longer had an immediate boss, but as blessings would have it, they had dismissed the Accounts Receivable person, and I was helping out with cash receipts, so my presence was still needed. Before long, I was in that Accounts Receivable position entirely. As I moved up the ranks, the more hours I worked, especially during my short time as the Office Manager by default. Another manager told me that I was going to work less now that I was getting a salary, suggesting I would take advantage of it, but it was quite the opposite. The company was drastically changing, from system software to policies and procedures, which contributed to me spending more time at the office. By all calculations, I was working for less per hour being a salaried employee than hourly. With my personality, this company had me on a string.

About 9:00 a.m. on Friday, August 6, 2001, I was getting into my morning routine at work when the phone rang. As I tried to complete the company's greeting, the person on the other end impatiently interrupted me mid welcome.

"Ma!" I recognized the voice of Mikey.

He was now in high school, and over the years, I seldom received a call from or about him from school, so naturally, my first reaction was of concern.

"What's wrong?" I answered, alarmed.

"Look at today's newspaper," demanded Mikey.

Chapter 6—Keep On Running

"Why?" I asked.

"Just look at it - I have to go. Bye."

Standing up from my chair, I hung up the phone and started towards my boss's office to see if he had the morning newspaper. Curiosity got its hold on me as I still thought something was wrong.

My boss did not have one that morning. Knowing that there was a convenience store across the street, I gave him a quick recap of my conversation with my son ending with, "Would you mind if I go across the street to get a paper." He agreed, and I quickly went back to my office for my purse and keys.

My heart was still slightly racing as I pushed open the glass door producing that familiar ring of the bell sounding the warning that someone had entered the store. Our City's newspaper, The Star-Banner, was stacked just a few feet from the front door. Approaching the stack, it became apparent without picking up the paper, the reason for the call.

On the front page to the right of the paper's logo banner was a picture of Mikey, clad in his blue and white sports attire as he jumped over a hurdle. My fear had instantly turned to pride, and my stern expression softened as a chuckle escaped my lips. "This is my son." I shared with the unconcerned cashier as she took my money for the newspaper, thinking I needed to explain my expression.

I was shocked as I read the story highlighting Mikey. as the Track and Field County champion in the 110-meter and 300-meter hurdles events. The embarrassing thing is, I did not know that he performed that event. Except for the weekend meet at the beginning of the season, I was too busy with work to attend his evening track meets.

The Cure Is In The Living

Since he was successful in the County event, he would progress to the District meet, so I requested the time off but still had a direct link to the office just in case they needed me.

I arrived late but got there before Mikey was lining up to run the 300-meter hurdles race; a lady sitting close by blurted out, "This is Mikey's race – another one for Belleview." Curious, I leaned over and introduced myself and asked what she meant by this is Mikey's race. "He has the best time all season; you have never seen him compete?"

I simply answered no and let the opinion fall where it may. Within seconds the gun was fired, and the race was in process. I was blown away by the ease and speed by which he scaled one hurdle after the other. Where have I been? How could I have missed this? In 39.5 seconds, Mikey crossed the finish line in first place. He was only .3 seconds from breaking the school record he had set earlier in the season. I never missed a track and field meet again, no matter the venue or the day of the week.

For a few months, I could feel a shift in the atmosphere at work when people from corporate started to visit our site. We were in the middle of a constitutional crisis due to errors made by top management from sheer ignorance of the rules. Company lawyers were interviewing every supervisor under them to accumulate the instructions passed down.

I was sitting in a conference room of a major hotel in Ocala early one Tuesday morning, dressed in a white quarter sleeve blouse neatly tucked into a black pencil skirt, black pantyhose, and heels. I was seated at the head of a large conference table facing four attorneys. I was not overly concerned since what I did was what I was told to do, and I had documentation of that. But my confidence changed when I

Chapter 6—Keep On Running

realized that my purpose there was not about my duties but what information I could share about someone else, which made me uncomfortable. In my evaluation, someone was either looking for a scapegoat or trying to protect him, but it was hard to figure out.

In the middle of questioning, one of the attorneys left the room to answer a telephone call. When she came back in, she asked for the recorder to stop and announced, "We won't be going home tonight; our flights are canceled." She was not able to finish before another asked, "Why?"

"Something about a plane crashing in the twin towers and the pentagon." It was the morning on Sept 11, 2001, and while I was living my life as a cancer survivor, over 2,900 lives ended at the hands of terrorists.

I worked long hours trying to make sure my work was getting done so that I had the time to support my child. One Thursday in particular as I was doing the end of month billing, the system was operating slowly, as it's known to do at times. I was scheduled to preach the following day, Good Friday, which was not a paid company holiday. I had to request the time off, so I did not want them to tell me I had to cancel it to complete billing, so I spent the entire night at the office working on billing. One of the staff members who became a dear friend over the years, decided to come back and spend part of the night with me so that I would not be alone. She left later to go home and prepare to return by 8:00 a.m.

As I sat there waiting for the computer to run the necessary reports, I had the strange feeling I was not going to be at that company for long. I started to pray out loud, asking the Lord that whatever the company was planning to do, to please hold off until after Mikey had completed the State championship, which was now only weeks away. His qualifying time for the 300 allowed him to compete at the State Meet to be held in Orlando, Florida. I did not want his first experience at State smeared with any degree of negativity.

As I was walking out of the office that Good Friday morning after being there for twenty-four hours, the staff coming in was puzzled when they noticed I was wearing the same clothes I had on the day before. I just waved goodbye, went home, took a shower, and slept for a few hours before getting up to review my Good Friday message to be delivered at one o'clock that afternoon.

The weekend came for Mikey to compete at the State championship. He ran his heat and was first as determined by a photo finish. He ran so hard that his heart was beating faster than he had ever experienced. "Ma, I thought my heart was going to burse, I will never run that hard again." I believe fear caused him a better position in the finals; he finished 3ʳᵈ fastest in the State of Florida that year.

I returned to work that Monday, and by Tuesday, claiming downsizing, I was laid off. God had answered my prayers, and that reality was more prominent than the lay off itself. There had been another set of layoffs previously, and I noticed one common factor; we had all invested in a profit-sharing offer made by the company years ago, and the maturity date was only months away. But for me, there was one additional element; I would have been vested for my pension within three days from the day they laid me off. I guess it was not all that bad; they did give back the amount I invested but not a penny more – they kept all the interest.

As I tried to find that ideal job, I worked as a domestic help during the day and watched over an older couple during the night filling in for people on vacation. The bills were coming in, and I needed to do my part. By the first an-

Chapter 6—Keep On Running

niversary of 911, I was working for an investment broker at a well-known investment firm. I was so miserable it was not funny – a salesperson I am not. It does not match my personality because I do not like rejection or confrontation. People were getting tired of phone solicitors, and we were at the crest of the National Do Not Call Registry. Not everyone is awestruck by a free meal offer, either. My primary function was to find attendees to "free" seminars in hopes of getting new clients.

The broker had high hopes for building her team, and she pushed for me to become a qualified agent. I failed that test miserably, it was not my thing, and I could not wrap my head around it. We both came to the same conclusion; the agent thing was not for me. What ended it for me though was reading an article in a local society magazine pointing out the lousy taste of a wealth manager who was handing out her business cards at a private event. It turned out to be my boss. Two weeks before Christmas, I was unemployed again.

My new job was a Manager's position at a relatively new company, but I stayed there only six weeks before my old boss from the garbage company asked for me to come to his office. He offered me the opportunity to go back to work for their newly formed company. I hesitated because I felt some obligation to the company I was working for, even though it was only a few weeks. I did not want them to think badly of me, but familiarity won, although it was not a management position. I knew the family well; I had a good relationship with them when I worked with them before. Not to mention, I would be three minutes away from my house again – I took the accounts receivable job.

As we grew, I became a supervisor over accounts receivable, and customer service and my unhealthy work habits started again. Things got so bad I would spend over 15 hours per day at times during the week and occasionally more hours during the weekend. My priorities now were work, church, and family and in that order. I still made it to choir practice, Bible Study, Prayer meeting, and kept up my secretarial duties, which included design and production of all programs for church events. My mom was not comfortable with computers, and had returned to school to pursue her Doctorate, so I became her typist and proofreader. Three hours of sleep was a good night.

I should have read the signs to slow down when occasionally I could feel the weakness in my legs at times when I stood up. But I kept pushing myself because I did not want to disappoint anyone.

Chapter 6—Keep On Running

A DREAM

Back on 3/1/2000, I had a dream. I was about to leave work and decided to call my children since I had not spoken to them all day. The phone was not a standard looking phone. The numbers were hard to dial and I had difficulty making the call. When I picked up the receiver again, I could hear my husband stating to a woman that yes, he still needed the place even if someone had reported the wrong address. He gave her the correct address as 5 Oak Run and confirmed that he would be moving on Nov 12.

I did not let on that I could hear the conversation but was in disbelief since we seemed to be doing fine. I was able to call and asked for the kids, and he told me they convinced him to leave them somewhere, so he did. I could see the two children he was referring to (a boy and a girl) like in a vision, and they were not my children because my two boys were in the room with my husband, who was on the phone with me.

I woke up from the dream concerned, so I wrote it down in a book.

The Cure Is In The Living

Chapter 7
Revelation of The Spot

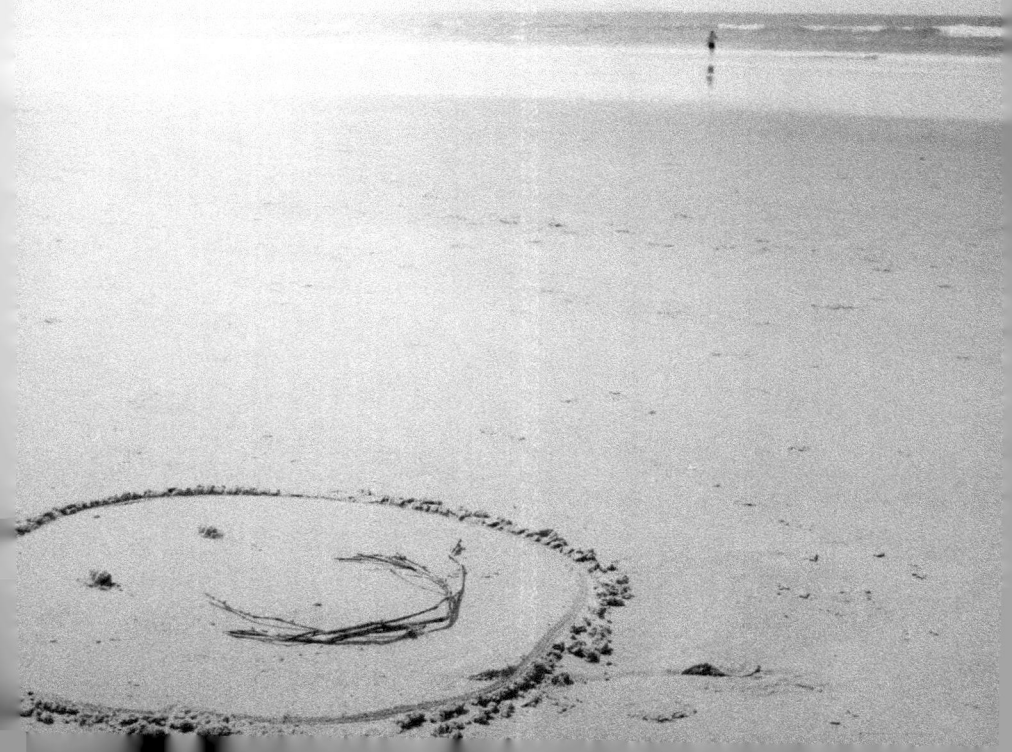

It was mid-day, and my mother called me at work "I was talking to a friend of mine today, and she told me about her daughter who was having chest pains but ignored it for a while. Eventually, when she went to the doctor, she found out she had suffered a mild heart attack. If you don't go to the hospital today, I am coming to take you." She threatened. Along with the occasional weak limbs, I had been complaining of an unusual intermittent sharp pain in my left chest. Whenever it occurred, it would stop me in my tracks but would pass within seconds. Since anxiety attacks were not strange for me, I assumed that was the case, especially since I was working such long hours between work and church. Home did not see me much.

Not wanting to find out that ignoring my mother's instructions could mean my life, I decided to go to the emergency room to get checked out. I left work early that evening and tried to find my son and husband to have them take me. I was not able to get their assistance, so I drove myself to the hospital and thought nothing of it except praying that they did not keep me overnight; there was work to be done.

As usual, the mention of chest pain put you ahead of everyone, and within minutes I had an IV going and several people asking me questions – then nothing. It was like hurrying up to wait. Alone I laid there waiting on some news when my mother and a church sister walked in to keep me company. Eventually, the doctors came back in to inform me that they did not find anything wrong with my heart, and discharge was imminent. However, before they let me go, they wanted to do a chest x-ray to see if I had a lung infection of sorts. "We just want to be sure before we send you home," I guess he repeated this for my peace of mind. I was taken to x-ray and back and waited. Eventually, he came in to tell me that they could see a spot on my left lung, and while he is not saying it is serious, he wanted me to contact my family doctor the following day and set an appointment to get it checked. "In fact, I will be leaving a message tonight for your doctor's office to call you to set the appointment as soon as possible. I don't want you to take this lightly." I drove myself back home..not feeling like talking to anyone since they did not think it was essential to accompany me to the hospital. That was my vindictive personality at play.

Before I could make the call, my doctor's office called me and set up the appointment for the following day. I liked my doctor; she was a simple, dainty middle-aged woman who did not act as if she was very materialistic. She always had on her white doctor's lab coat with visible long time wear.

She made her diagnosis and ordered a PET scan and 30 days of antibiotics to treat for possible infection as she was treating an otherwise healthy 46 years old female who had never smoked.

I was too busy with all I had to do to be scared and kept up my heavy schedule. The company being in the middle of a significant system conversion, which was testing everybody's nerves, demanded already long days to be longer. I was still typing a Thesis along with my Church duties, which also included preaching twice per month. Nevertheless, I was reminded of the condition each time I experience that sharp pain in the left side of my chest. Yet I remained fearless because I felt it was nothing, and the medication would take care of whatever was ailing me - the spot would be a thing of the past when they recheck.

The end of October completed treatment and another scan taken; the spot did not change. I still was not moved by it and simply would comply with the next step, which was the referral to a Pulmonologist.

Chapter 7—Revelation of the Spot

When I got home that evening, I gave my husband the doctor's findings and recommendations. "They are going to do a biopsy to see what it is" I concluded

"Ok," he responded.

Things were very strained between my husband and me by then – no one was happy, and the idea of divorce had already left the starting line. So such an answer did not bother me. The following week I left work a little earlier than usual to take the family out for dinner to celebrate his birthday as I was trying to keep it as sane as possible for the boys.

I cannot recall what happened that caused us to sit down together on Nov 18, 2006, a week after his birthday. However, we had a heart to heart, and at the end I said. "We have been at this for a long time. Let's forget about this divorce thing and focus on our family." And he agreed.

Looking back, I am not sure what he agreed to, because the following day, he left not only the home but the State to start a new life and a new family. It was the beginning of the end of a 22 year 11 months, and three (3) days marriage.

The dream I had six years ago on March 1, 2000 was now revealed. My husband left without saying anything to anyone on Nov 19, 2006, while the boys and I were at church. I believe the reason why he did not move on the 12th as stated in the dream was because that Sunday, I was too ill to go to church, so I stayed home, something as rare as a child saying no to candy. The woman he left me for had a daughter and a son.

The Cure Is In The Living

Chapter 8

The Biopsy

My consulting appointment with the Pulmonologist started with a battery of lung tests. I inhaled and exhaled at different speeds through different mouthpieces as they measured the amount and rate of air I was breathing. Then there were comparisons with non-medicated and medicated results. The tests were very intense, and I found myself having to take a breather now and then. It was one instruction after another; hold your breath for a while and push the air out quickly – then empty your lungs fully – this time, breathe normally. It actually took your breath away at times.

In a couple of weeks, I was back at the doctor's office for the results. With my attention directed to x-ray images of my lung clipped to some dimly lit boxes, the doctor translated the results. All I heard were percentages and measurements until the conclusion that they did not find any other problems with my lungs, making biopsy the next step.

My first option, they could go down my nose, but there was a strong possibility of missing the location of the mass and producing healthy tissue instead. Second, go through my side, using a needle guided procedure. In this instance, the possibility of missing the spot is less, but it could collapse my lung. And third, open my chest.

This doctor's appointment was no different for me. Here I was alone with a big decision on the table. I had no idea what to do, so I asked for some extra time to think about it. He was concluding the office visit when I happened to ask if the 80% lung capacity was normal range. "No," the doctor replied with no follow-up explanation.

For some reason, I was disappointed, not because of the number but because this bit of additional information was not shared. As the expert, why wasn't he more forthcoming with the details of my condition? What other information hadn't he shared that would help me decide the type of treatment that would be best? As the patient, not necessarily knowing what normal lung capacity was, I should not have to ask. Going forward, trusting him was daunting. So I requested a 2nd opinion, and he gave me the name of another doctor.

What I did not realize was that he did not actually give me someone for a second opinion but instead had referred me to the surgeon. It worked out well anyway. Dr. Chandra had a kind and patient mannerism and explained the procedures clearly. Dr. Chandra claimed to be the only doctor in the area who was practicing a method that would pinpoint the exact location of the mass - this improved accuracy for testing the affected area. The procedure would require a three day recovery period, which was ok with me. My concerns were at rest.

Still focusing on being positive and exercising faith that this was not cancer, I was still sensitive to the fact that it could be so. This reality did not minimize my trust in what God could do here; in fact, he could choose for it to be cancer. I was practical and told Dr. Chandra that if it turns out to be cancer, do not wait to tell me but go ahead and do what needs to be done and remove it. And he agreed.

It was now the beginning of December and months since the initial findings, so imagine my surprise when the scheduler from his office called to set the appointment and gave me options still weeks away. I chose the earliest, which was within a month. Everyone knowledgeable of the situation was not showing much urgency or concern, which fed my confidence that I would be ok.

My time off request was for three days. All my work schedules and assignments going forward were planned around me returning in three days – it is not cancer - I will be back in three days. That was my belief, and I was sticking to it.

Chapter 8—The Biopsy

The day of reckoning came; it was January 31, 2007, and the biopsy was scheduled for 8:00 a.m. that morning. I took my second shower with the special antibacterial soap they had given me. It was cold that morning. By Ocala standards, that would be mid-fifties. Therefore, a sweater would be necessary for the short five-mile ride. Before long, my mom arrived to take me to the hospital. Dressed in my burnt orange mid-length sweater trimmed with brown piping and jeans, I gathered my overnight bag and purse and headed out the door into the dark chilled atmosphere.

By 6:00 a.m., I was walking into admissions with the same two people who were in that emergency room when the spot was first discovered - my mother and a member of our church. My oldest son Mikey had come home from college the night before, so he and Nathan would join them later that morning. I do not believe that at any time since this started, did I wonder how my children were feeling; it never entered my mind. Yet, everything for work and church was set for my three-day absence.

Still as calm as I could be, the registration process was complete, and I was taken by wheelchair upstairs to another holding area. With hospital garb on, I waited to get the needle inserted to mark the spot on my lung. After a while, a young lady appeared with her stretcher and told me she was taking me down to get an x-ray. I understood enough to know that a CT scan and an x-ray were completely two different things. It sounded odd to me, so I asked, "Is this going to be a regular x-ray?"

"One was ordered," she replied.

"Ok, but what I am asking is, are you taking me down just to x-ray my chest? Because... if that is the intent that is not the procedure I should be having," I said reluctantly.

She was just the transporter, of course, so she left the

The Cure Is In The Living

room to consult with the nurse. I could see the puzzled look on my mom's face since she had no idea why I would be disputing the order. "What the doctor told me was, they are to have a wire inserted through my side to the place where the spot is located, guided by a CT scan; it's not an x-ray," I explained, defending my actions.

The transporter came back with the nurse, and I told her the same thing outlining my doctor's orders, and if that is where this young lady is taking me, then yes. If not, please call the doctor to confirm the order.

We could hear a couple of nurses arguing down the hall trying to decipher the doctor's order - it seems as if it was a matter of interpretation. I got off my stretcher and clutched the back of my crumbled green and off white hospital gown, and walked to the nurse's station. "I am sorry, but why don't you simply call the doctor? He explained the procedure to me, and I am sure it is not just an x-ray." I asserted.

A few minutes later, a nurse came in trying to be upbeat and positive and confirmed that I was correct. "they left off one word from the order, so we did not know.." I interrupted her before she could finish her sentence, "So what are we doing now?" I questioned.

Her answer matched what the doctor had told me needed to be done, except now we were running behind. The radiologist who did the procedures had completed his rounds at the hospital and had already left for his office. "But, He is on his way back," she said, and left the room.

I recognized the large doughnut-shaped base with its long narrow motorized table to be the CT scanner as I was wheeled into the room. Glad I would not be here long because that table was hard, with absolutely no cushioning. But to be honest, my other reason for not liking this machine is

Chapter 8—The Biopsy

because I am claustrophobic, and the long tube or doughnut shape, which they call the open version, did not make a difference to me. As long as it surrounds me, I still feel trapped when my face is within the area of the base. Quickly the radiologist came into the room and gave me a few instructions and adjusted my gown to expose the side just below my left armpit – he was ready to start.

He told me I was about to feel a slight sting, some pressure, and a bit of discomfort as he inserted the wire through my side and towards my lung. He further explained that the procedure was divided into three steps. He will make the first entry, go back to the booth and scan to determine the position, and repeat it until the wire is positioned by the affected tissue. I said ok and took a deep breath.

Oh yes, empathetically, you are probably feeling right now what I felt then; the first push was not just discomfort; it was a pain. The doctor switched places with an attendant, covered with protective wear, as he went back to the booth to examine his handy work. The assistant was to be my assurance that I was doing fine and to make sure I did not move. "It is important that you do not move as we put you in to take a picture of the site. I'm going to be right over there if you need me," the assistant said, hesitating to make sure I acknowledged his instructions.

I was not interested in where 'over there' was. I was in disbelief that this thing was so painful. But if I stop now, I will have to start over, so let's keep going. Don't complain; it must be me, you can do it, be strong. I told myself.

"You are doing good, Mrs. Morris," came the voice through the microphone as the table exited the base of the CT scan machine. The attendant reappeared, followed by the doctor.

By the end of the second push, it was downright painful. My mind was all over the place. *I am strong; I can bear this. They could not have known the degree of pain. It must be me. Be strong. You can do this.* I tried to focus as I kept whispering the name of Jesus. "Breath, you are doing well," I heard from a voice somewhere in the room, "But.. it's... hard," I responded between labored breaths.

As the attendant attempted to console me, he lifted his left hand to place it on my shoulder, and immediately I recognized his ring. He was the same guy who did my CT scan at the hospital weeks prior." What was so unique that I recognized the ring so quickly and not the person's face that I had been looking at for several minutes? On his ring finger was a simple broad gold band with a clearly outlined cross.

I viewed that tiny cross as a message that the Lord was with me. I found new strength - *I can do this. Breathe, Barbara, breathe. It's not going to last forever. Hold on and breathe. My gaze was on that ring until the assistant had to give way to the doctor for the third push on the wire. The discomfort, as they call it, got worse with every insertion, as was apparent by the tears falling down my cheeks. It is funny to think that before this, I often ridiculed the exaggeration of the words "it's like an elephant sitting on my chest," but I qualified that day to use those words: it felt like some ridiculous amount of pressure. Each time I inhaled, it was like trying to push heavy weights using weak unconditioned muscles. "This cannot be real, Lord, please help me." By now, my cry to my heavenly Father was tapered but just beyond a whisper.*

The monster of the day came back to inform me that it's done and secured the wire as a few more guys entered the room, casually talking to each other. I remember the doctor telling them to hurry up with just a hint of urgency in his

Chapter 8—The Biopsy

voice. They continued to converse as they escorted me down the hall with no care in the world while I kept calling on the name of Jesus to help me. I was in tears from the pain and the heaviness in my chest and wanted desperately to stop feeling.

They transported me just a short distance to another room, accompanied by the radiology assistant, and handed over to another team. As the assistant relayed my previous whereabouts and handed over my chart, the new guy glanced at it and asked, "what did you give her – I don't see it written here."

"We did not give her anything," was the reply.

The new guy moved swiftly to check my heartbeat as he continued in disbelief "you did the procedure without giving her anything?" he questioned with obvious concern.

"Yes." The assistant responded and walked away.

My new team member, now my hero, called out, and a young lady walked quickly towards him as he blurted out a doctor's name for her to call. I guess she was not moving as fast as the situation dictated because, within seconds, he repeated his instructions, this time with more urgency as he added the words "STAT...her heart rate is...." lights out!

When they revived me, I was in another location with two new faces. "Hi Mrs. Morris, how are you doing? We are going to take you to surgery now." One of them said in his polite and caring voice. I could not respond at first because I was trying to figure out where I was and what had happened. The first reality was that the pain in my chest was gone, and an IV was attached to my arm. With that observation, I answered yes to the question.

"Good, we are taking you to surgery now," he repeated as I was scouting the room, and the stretcher started to move. I could see people in dark green scrubs and covered heads with masks hanging with only two of the four strings securing it around their necks.

The ride ended rather quickly as I was in the operating room now, with its big round lamps extending from the ceiling and trays draped with crisp blue paper and multiple shiny instruments on display. The room appeared to be empty despite the presence of several monitors and attendants. The foot of the operating table was towards the door, so I could hear a few 'hellos' intended for me echoing from different directions of the room, but the greeting that got my attention was a woman who entered the room as if she was in charge. I could see her clearly as she walked straight over to me. With no evaluation at all, she said, "we can remove this and get her ready," as she reached for the drape covering my left side.

It took nothing for me to holler back, "No, there is a wire there in my side, please be careful."

"There is?" she asked in surprise as she stopped herself from yanking the sheet of paper. Gently she raised it and responded, "Oh," as she put the yellow sheet back and disappeared behind me. It was like an 'oops' without the acknowledgment of stupidity.

Unbeknownst to everyone, that thin piece of wire was linked to my assurance that when this was all over, they would have tested the exact area, significantly reducing the chance for error. It would be clear, leaving no doubt of cancer. Plus, I already paid the price of having it inserted – I was not about to go through that pain again. Will, somebody give me an amen? (Side note: I learned from the surgery notes that the wire did get dislodged before the surgeon got there.)

Chapter 8—The Biopsy

The plan of the morning was a "Thoracoscopy and biopsy. Possible open lung biopsy. Possible lobectomy." Jesus, I'm in your care," was my prayer before I started to count..100, 99, 98, 97, 96, 95...

The Cure Is In The Living

Chapter 9

The "C" Diagnosis

I was on the move when I gained consciousness while they were taking me to the Surgical Intensive Care Unit. Severe discomfort was present on my left side, but I did not quite put it together until a voice from my right called my name. Looking toward the voice, I realized it was my mother.

Apparently, my action assured her that I was awake and coherent enough to comprehend her words that followed; "it is cancer." They were the three words I did not want to hear, but the reality was about to change my course for the rest of my life. No exaggeration intended.

It is strange the things we think of during a crisis. The first thought that entered my mind was that I was going to lose my hair. No, it was not vanity at all, so let me help you to see it from my perspective. You see, five years earlier I had cut my hair, reducing it from a length beyond my shoulders to about 2 inches from my scalp. But with my busy lifestyle, It did not take long for me to miss the days I could gather my hair into a ponytail. For that reason, I would often vow to God that I would not cut my hair off like that again. Now it's all grown back, and even longer than before, I was going to lose it all anyway. I actually chuckled silently, considering the irony of it all.

I became stationary again, and a few people around my bed. My mother's voice is the only one I remember as she proclaimed how good God is. Apparently, because my lungs had fully collapsed during surgery, they told my family not to be frightened when they saw me because I might be on a respirator. It just so happened that I was not. My lungs did what it needed to do, and I was breathing fully on my own. It was now after 5:00 p.m. – the scheduled 8:00 a.m. procedure did not end until after 4:00 p.m.

The Cure Is In The Living

By the following morning, I was experiencing the full repercussion from the eight-inch incision. It started from my side, a few inches under my arm, going in the direction towards the center of my back, then curving slightly upwards at the bra line. This skillful cutting through skin, flesh, and muscle had allowed entry to my left lung through the bed of my sixth rib.

Now there I was, lying helplessly, my head scooted off the pillow and just inches from having an encounter with the bedrail. I could not find the strength to pull my torso towards the center of the bed. A wave of hopelessness came over me as my multiple attempts failed. Being brave and independent was not my intent right now. That behavior had gone out the door a long time ago. The fact was I could not seem to get anyone's attention to help me. With all sorts of tubes attached to and in me, accidentally dislodging any of them would have been catastrophic to me. I have accepted that tubes inserted while sedated are the best kind.

You might not have experienced this personally, but most likely have seen those advertisements where an older adult has fallen and unable to get up, and they are all alone; that is how I felt. Except there should be someone close or a call button in reach. I worked in hospitals for years, and I know the rules.

The Surgical Intensive Care Unit had curtained cubicles with a nurse's station in the center of the unit, yet no one was in sight from my viewpoint. As I adjusted my left hand, I noticed a saline-soaked bandage and blood backing up into the IV tube - another desperate visual sweep of the room yielded nothing. With my IV leaking, experiencing sharp pain, feeling helpless and alone, the tears flowed uncontrollably. "Lord, I know you are with me wherever I go. Please, Lord, send help," I prayed.

Chapter 9—The "C" Diagnoses

The first doctor to visit that morning was the Pulmonologist I had seen outside the hospital. I honestly thought he was out of the picture after giving me the referral, but here he was to validate collecting the hospital visit fee. This time, however, he earned a few brownie points because following behind him was my nurse, who I am sure was nervous since he had not checked on me for a while. Without knowing it, the doctor had brought me the help I needed. By the end of his visit, he had duplicated my mother's words from the night before that I had cancer.

Having the nurse's attention, at last, I spewed out all my needs before he left the room. He made note that my vein housing the IV needle was no longer useful and that he would change the site in a minute. His first order of business would be to consult with the doctor to get the pain under control since the epidural I had for pain management was not working. He was sure to stress that I should not hesitate to inform them immediately if I was in pain to adjust medication. All I could think was, Is he serious right now? I have been trying to do just that since I woke up and could not find anyone to listen to me.

Despite my condition, though, I had heard enough about addiction to pain meds, so I voiced my concern. He explained that for the next few days, we run the risk of a collapsed lung if I am not breathing to extend my lungs fully. The probability of that happening will increase if I am not breathing well due to the pain.

"We are monitoring you closely; you don't have to worry about addiction. Right now, we need you to breathe." His summary made perfect sense, so who was I to argue – bring it on. After several hours and a few attempts, they figured morphine was not working, so Dilaudid and Toradol became my pain relief cocktail.

The Cure Is In The Living

There was an older man in the cubicle next to me, and I overheard him saying to his visitor that she should not worry because he had beaten it twice before, and he will do it again. His words gave me a flicker of hope – this might not be the end for me, after all. This bit of hope increased when my General Practitioner came in to do her rounds.

"So it's cancer after all," I said to her.

"We don't know that as yet," she replied, indicating that they were still waiting on the Pathology report.

"But they said it is cancer," I replied, puzzled.

She inquired who gave me that information because it was not conclusive, according to the reports. *She read from the paper in her hand, 'Pathology is still pending.'*

"Is it possible everyone else was wrong?" was the thought running through my mind. I know a God who could make it possible. But it would not be so. The hint of hope she brought did not last past the next doctor to visit.

The hospital pulmonologist assigned to me entered my small cubicle and stood at the foot of my bed for a few seconds with his hands on his hips and a puzzled look on his face as he looked at me. This visit was my first time meeting him, but he seemed to be a light-hearted sort of a fellow. He confirmed that I was who I was supposed to be as he walked closer to the side of the bed.

"Except for your bed hair, you look great. You do not look like someone who went through your type of surgery less than 24 hours ago," the Doc said in amazement.

I mustered a smile and a faint thank you as he continued to explain a few things while he checked me over, listening to my heart and lungs, the standard stuff that doctors do. Looking behind me, he asked if I was using the incentive spirometer. I followed his pointing finger to an apparatus on the table a ways off behind me.

Chapter 9—The "C" Diagnoses

He was referring to the hollow clear plastic chamber with a blue accordion-like tube having one end attached to the chamber and a mouthpiece at the other end. The chamber was divided into two unequal parts. On the smaller side within the chamber housed a yellow ball, and on the larger side of the air chamber were markings of different levels and an indicator. I had no idea it was there for my use. Although it was within my curtained area, it was far enough away from the bed that I wondered if it was left there after the previous patient. We all know my luck; I was not leaving it up to chance.

He received his answer from the expression on my face because he continued to point out the importance of using an incentive spirometer to strengthen my lungs and prevent unwanted lung issues that can occur after surgery. I acknowledged all he had to say, and he left, leaving me still hopeful that I just might make it out of this unscathed. My faith was at a place where I believed despite what it looked like, there could still be a miracle. But, there comes a time when it is what it is, and the diagnosis was official - I had Stage 1 non-small cell Adenocarcinoma. The sucker had been identified.

The Cure Is In The Living

Chapter 10

The Beginning of Recovery

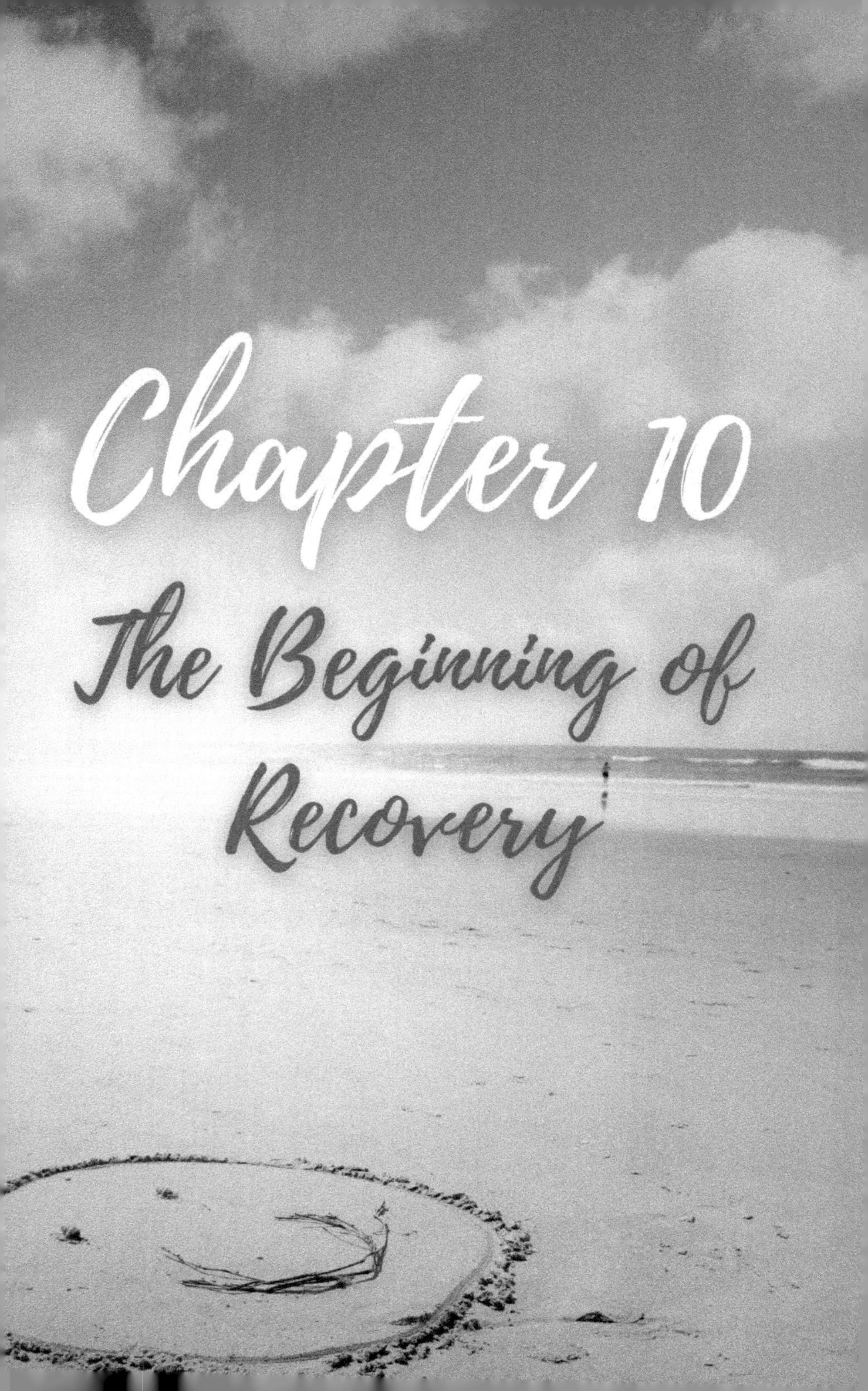

Chapter 10—The Beginning of Recovery

By the middle of day one post-operative, the pain had subsided enough for me to start using the spirometer but not before requesting a new one. Of course, I made sure the existing one was still there behind me when they brought in the new one just in case. Hey, I have heard enough stories to be cautious, and I needed to make sure they did not take the one from the room and bring the same one back. With my luck, who knows.

By day two, the need to cough was great and utterly painful. Yet everyone kept telling me that I needed to cough. To this day, I cannot see the benefit of holding a pillow in trying to accomplish that task when the stapled incision was in my back. The area felt tight and sore. I envisioned it to be like a turkey stuffed and sewed up, and as it cooks in the oven, the skin pulls apart. What if my stitches came undone? Why didn't anyone understand my fears?

I was affixed with a patient-controlled analgesia pump administering the Dilaudid medication. From a patient's point of view, this is quite misleading. "Whenever you feel the pain coming, press this button for the pain medication," they told me. What is not usually explained is that while the pump is set to give the pain medication upon command, there is still a limit as to how much medicine I can get regardless of how many times I press that button.

My dosage never seemed to last as long as it should before the pain came back, and so sleeping was a problem. I would finally fall asleep; then the pain started. It would take some time to go back to sleep just to start the process over again. We eventually found out that the medicine was in one-hour increments only. So, Nathan had the bright idea, one I think he enjoyed too much.

My son witnessing my discomfort and pain took the control button from me. He methodically watched that clock, and each time the clock reached that one hour mark, he would press that button for his mother so that she could rest. He became my official medicine administrator that day and was very proud of it. That was the only way I was able to sleep. A time of not knowing where I was and what had happened to me, nor did I have to think of what was to come. Sleep was an escape from my unknown reality – if even just for a few hours.

It was a struggle for them to get me to a chair by day three, and my nurse was very annoyed with 'my poor effort to move.' I do not know what her specialty was, but she kept complaining that she was the only one of her caliber on the floor and felt the patient-to-nurse ratio was unfair. She was noticeably overweight, could have been in her early sixties, and seemed sort of edgy and unfocused. I had not been out of bed since surgery as required. The doctor was coming to do rounds and she expressed this concern, but I did not acknowledged her. So, she repeated herself.

"The doctor is planning on taking the tubes out today, and I need to get you out of bed and seated in that chair now," she said, almost complaining about the pending task. I had two drainage tubes from my back and catheters emptying into a few reservoirs hanging from my bed, an IV in my arm, and still had a fear of something coming loose - and they wanted me to do what? Moving just did not seem possible – to me. But as you would imagine, the nurse won the argument.

After some struggle and a long five minutes of me trying to move myself with minimal assistance, I had made my first steps since surgery and was sitting in a chair with all my mechanisms intact. For me, it was one small step today; the giant leap can wait for next week. If truth be told, I desired and needed a shower more than sitting in that chair.

Chapter 10—The Beginning of Recovery

My anxious nurse was correct as the doctor was present a couple of hours later to remove the tubes. We now had two eager people in the room, a nurse trying her best to please the doctor and me, the victim who did not know what to expect. The feeling experienced as the tube was pulled out is one that I cannot put in words. I was just thankful when it was over and the opening sutured. The next order of business was another chest x-ray to secure my move to the Progressive Care unit. The x-ray showed a 10% pneumothorax, which meant an abnormal collection of air in the space between the lung and the chest wall. Assured that the percentage was not that abnormal and can go away within days gave me some comfort.

It was now late afternoon, and the nurse's shift was coming to an end. She had one more task to complete our day's encounter and that was to take me to my new location. My sons and my mother had arrived by the time the nurse came by with a wheelchair. It was a rush to take me to my new abode. My sons left the room to wait by the door to join the entourage when we came out. At a snail's pace, I tried to lift myself out of the reclining chair with the use of only my right arm. I was not moving fast enough, so my annoyed nurse, expressing her lack of patience, uttered, "We need to get going, let me help you," as she tucked both her hands under my left arm.

Everyone inside and outside the unit heard my scream. It's often said that a child knows their mother's voice, and I proved it that day. My sons came running and pulled the curtain back just to hear my words, "That's the side where I had the surgery." If looks could kill, that poor nurse would be on the floor twice over. "Are you crazy?" I heard Nathan's voice followed simultaneously by Mikey, "Mom! you ok?"

The Cure Is In The Living

The nurse, obviously shaken from her mistake and the eyewitnesses to her behavior kept apologizing and trying to explain herself on the trip over. Still, no one was making her feel better. The word sorry is easily said but never takes away the initial pain caused by our actions. I did not dislike her, but I thought retirement might not be a bad idea.

My next morning in a private room in the Progressive Care unit was surprisingly better than my past few days. A shower was not recommended, but I came as close to it as possible with the help of a nurse's aide. I replaced the hospital gown with my mint green pajamas embellished with pink roses on the lapels and pockets. A lot of thought went into purchasing my hospital ensemble. I had to be sure that my medical team would have easy access for examination and quick removal if it became necessary. Hence, they were a bigger size than necessary and short sleeves so that my IV was always visible. Even the pockets worked out fine as a place to house the heart monitor, which had become a typical protocol so that I could be monitored from outside the room.

I always went into the hospital with my personal sleepwear. So getting out of the hospital gown felt so exhilarating. For as long as I could remember, my mother had a drawer with washed, pressed, and neatly folded sleepwear if a trip to the hospital was necessary. Oh, I forgot to add, new underwear was also a necessity. I had such a dresser drawer up to the time I left Jamaica for the United States and simply did not keep up the tradition. But, having new 'nighties' (as we refer to everything that we sleep in) to take to the hospital was still a tradition worth upholding.

Shortly after breakfast on day four, I got myself up out of the chair, put on my pink floral silk robe, and off I went down the hall with my IV pole. That leap was nearer than I initially thought. I was starting to feel more energetic,

Chapter 10—The Beginning of Recovery

not only in my body but also in my emotional state. I refused to think of tomorrow, telling myself, *"God has it already laid out for me and whatever it is, I will just have to embrace it. For right now, I need to be healthy again, and if I keep walking as much as possible, that will happen."*

Day five post-operative, and if all went well, the discharge was hours away. My doctor's assistant came by and told me she was going to order a chest x-ray to make sure the pneumothorax, which was still present, had not increased further than the day before. However, when the nurse came in, she told me to contact the person who will be taking me home because the discharge order was processed. I inquired about the chest x-ray. She left the room to check on the order, but soon after returned quite abruptly. She repeated the discharge order and informed me that an x-ray was not required. She did not take kindly to my persistent questioning and once again told me to make the telephone call for someone to get me within the next 2 hours.

I was released into the care of my mother, where I intended to stay for the next week until I could take care of myself. Mikey had gone back to college, and Nathan, who was preparing to conclude his High School senior year, was the only one I had at home at this point.

For the next few days, I found myself crying. With the Darvocet, Morphine sulfate extended-release tablets, and over the counter ibuprofen to be taken in-between the prescription meds (if needed), I had enough medication to dull the physical pain. That was not the reason for the rocky emotions. Instead, reality was setting in. I looked for answers to the why, what, and how long questions as they raced through my thoughts like race cars zooming by on a racetrack. I did not have the strength or know it all to answer one question before the other came whooshing by.

The Cure Is In The Living

Within a few days of discharge, my sister arrived from Virginia to help with my care. It was the help that I did not realize beforehand that would, well – be helpful. I had strange experiences after surgery. The weirdest of them all, scratching an itch on my side and feeling the sensation on my thigh. This freaked – me – out! It was an itch I could not seem to scratch.

Although my surgery was on my left side, it did not occur to me that trying to use my right would be an issue, but I found out otherwise very quickly the first time I tried to reach behind me. Surprise! Somehow, the left muscles also became engaged in that movement. I needed help to take a shower because I still needed to keep the surgical areas dry, and I could not hold my hand above the head nor reach behind me without feeling a tug on the left side. Lifting my legs to get over the tub was also a challenge. Although challenging, these tasks should not cause the pain I had now developed in the chest each time I breathe. It caused enough concern that I called the doctor to report the problem. She instructed me to go to the radiologist for a chest x-ray to have a look at the area.

My sister believes that a sure-fire way for a woman to feel revived is to get her hair and nails done, so she offered to take her ailing sister to Radiology and then to get a wash and blow in hopes of lifting my spirits. X-ray complete, we set off to Fantastic Sams, which was approximately ten minutes away from the Radiology office. When we got to the hair salon, the young lady who approached us had to be informed of my situation for overall understanding. Then came the specifics of limited mobility, no sudden jerks or adjustments, and being extra gentle. That was easy for her, but the challenge was her familiarity, or lack thereof, with my African hair type. Of course, we were a walk-in, so we assured her that she could do it since all we needed was a wash, blow-dry, and flat iron - that should work for all hair types.

She struggled with the wash as she mentioned that my hair is so thick, but she managed to get through it and onto the blow-out. As she toiled at that as well, my sister received a call from my mom stating that my doctor's office had called several times, wanting me to call them back immediately. The telephone call was a saving grace for me because I was starting to hurt, and for my hairstylist, because we no longer had the time to get the straightening done. She hurried through the remainder of the drying process and scooped it all into a ponytail, and out the door we went.

We got to the car and made the phone call to the doctor's office. The office manager was very annoyed at me for not calling back immediately and explained that they received the results from the x-ray, and the pneumothorax had increased in size to the point that I needed to be readmitted. Anger came before fear because of one reason. Remember the day of discharge when I tried to convince them that the x-ray of my lungs was needed before I left to make sure the pneumothorax had not increased? Well, here we are.

As I started to complain, the office manager interrupted, "Which hospital would you like to go to?"

I gave her the name of the hospital but also inquired what that readmission meant for me. She transferred me to the doctor, who explained that it's possible that they might have to put the tube back in if it does not decrease on its own. They had already notified the surgeon who would make the ultimate decision, but it had increased enough to warrant being watched by the professionals. I hung up the phone, still complaining to my sister how this could have been avoided. The stress was not helping; it was only making my breathing worse.

The Cure Is In The Living

We went back to my mother's to pick her up and get my hospital bag to head to the hospital. Upon arrival at the hospital, my attitude did not change one iota. I was now dealing with a co-pay; I did not have money to pay. I had gone into that hospital with the intent of a biopsy, and a few days recovery to a full-blown open rib surgery and financial status was not something I wanted to handle at that time. My sister jumped in, trying to help with getting alternative options. I have been in an upright position now since mid-morning, missed my afternoon meds, and the pain was getting sharper. I was growing tired, so as they kept going back and forth about the co-pay, I lost it. "Can't all this wait? I just need to lay down right now; can you please get me to a room," I said, raising my voice. Yes, I was angry at the hospital because I should not be dealing with this right now.

Fear had returned, not knowing what the pocket of air could be doing to my health. Get me hooked up to something, I needed the pain to stop, and I needed them to start figuring out a way to correct the problem before it got worse.

I identified the pain to be similar to labor contractions. The pain starts and builds in intensity, then gets to the peak, stays there for a couple of seconds, and then subside. After several minutes it starts over again. And that is how I explained it to my sister, my mother, and every nurse when asked to describe the pain. It was late evening when the surgeon came in, puzzled that I was back in the hospital. To him, I described the pain as waves thinking that he could not fully comprehend my experience if I used the labor contractions description. My conversation was interrupted by, "You have been complaining that it is like contractions, and now the doctor is here you are saying it is like waves." Having been at the brink of 'closing my eyes' and in a 'not care about what happens next' mentality for a while now, I stopped talking. I allowed everyone else to answer the questions as to what had happened. The doctor caught on as he walked closer, looked directly at me, and asked me a few more 'yes' or 'no' questions before leaving the room.

Pain management was still an issue because I found it difficult to sleep as the pain escalated, so OxyContin became the next choice. It would knock me out within seconds of it entering my vein. From the first dose, it was apparent that this drug made me incoherent. Although I hold no secret that will bring down a nation, I made a conscious decision not to answer any questions or engage in conversation once I felt the drug's effects within a matter of seconds. I found the drug that helped control the pain for hours and would often ask for it. However, the number of times I was allowed to have it was limited not only to a per-hour regimen but per my hospital stay, so they spaced out the doses.

No one had to prompt me this time to get out of bed, though. Walking was now my natural medicine. If I keep walking, my lungs will get stronger, and if my lungs get stronger, I will get better faster. I intended to do everything I could do to ensure that I get better. God was faithful to me once again because I did not have to do another surgical procedure. Within a few days, the pneumothorax had decreased, and I was rid of the hospital - but not for long.

It was time for the first follow-up at the doctor's office, and for the second time in my adult life, I got dressed and left my home without wearing a bra. The incision ran just above the base of my bra lines, making it impossible to wear one painlessly.

Mikey was back in town to drive me to my appointment since Nathan was in school, preparing for finals. The ride there was uneventful. It was filled with gratitude as I was thankful to drive down the familiar streets and see the stores and landmarks – things that otherwise did not get my attention. Right then, I was alive, and I felt thankful.

Sitting there in the doctor's waiting room in my spacious yellow top and denim skirt, I felt as if everyone knew I was not appropriately dressed. So as much as I could, I folded my arms across my chest with my right hand resting in the crease by my left elbow while resting the left hand on my right shoulder. The camouflage was perfect – as if anyone noticed. The devastating truth is, it was all in my mind being concerned about how others saw me instead of what I am. My girls were not big swingers, so they were not noticeable at all. Yet, it concerned me enough to mention it to the doctor. I needed help in knowing what other patients who have been in my situation had done. His assistant gave me a few options and sent me off to Victoria's Secret with specific instructions to provide the sales attendant there who will know exactly what I needed. Our next stop was Victoria's Secret, then to my workplace to pick up my paychecks and back home.

We were just getting home and walking through the door to a ringing phone. Running had become a thing of the past, for now. So I walked as fast as I could to get the phone. As I leaned over to pick it up and straighten up again, I felt as if something shifted on my lower left side. It was not painful but uncomfortable, so I massaged the area slightly, tried to breathe through it, and continued through the afternoon. I was resting when Mikey came to say he was leaving; he had to go back for classes the next day.

As night time approached, the contraction type of pain I had shortly after my first discharge from the hospital had returned, but the location was a few inches lower than before.

Chapter 10—The Beginning of Recovery

I remained in bed thinking I overdid it. The time-release morphine dulled the pain some, but I could still feel the annoying sensation. About one o'clock the following morning, I was awakened by the need to use the bathroom. A sharp pain from that same spot hindered my first attempt to move. My second attempt proved the same result; the morphine had lost its grip on this pain.

I remained still for a second. "Well, if I wet the bed, only I would know. Nah, with my luck, I might need someone to help me, then my accident would no longer be a secret, so get up, you can do it." I said aloud.

"Breath B, breath through it," I encouraged myself. But nothing was working, so I called out to Nathan. I waited a minute, and my fear was confirmed. I could not raise my voice loud enough to wake someone in a deep sleep on the opposite side of the house – he did not hear me. I tried again to get out of the bed – if only I could turn over, I can do this. Nope, it's not happening. Maybe he will hear the cell phone. My cell phone was always on the bed, so it was reachable without much effort. I called, and thank God he answered. I explained my dilemma, and he came over noticeably not happy having to get up at this hour. He tried to help lift my upper body out of bed, but the pain was too much. He then rolled me onto my side, holding both my legs and pulled them off the bed first before lifting me into a standing position.

Gingerly, I walked to the bathroom, but as I tried to sit on the toilet, the pain was so excruciating that I momentarily lost my sight. I was conscious, but everything was complete darkness. Having a wire pierce my side and into my lungs without anesthesia was a cake walk to this pain. There was nothing to grasp, so I planted my hands against the shower door to my right to stabilize myself and called out, "Oh Jesus - help me!"

The cry was hardly out of my mouth before my sight came back, but the urge to urinate had increased, and I could not bend at the waist. Having my son either come in to help me sit or clean up after me was not about to happen. It's a good thing that my imagination was still working. With tiny steps and shallow breaths, I turned around to face the toilet, moved forward so that I was standing directly over the toilet bowl, and let her rip while standing up. That turned out to be much more comfortable than the challenge that followed to try and redress myself. "God, why didn't you bless me with a daughter as well?" I thought.

With baby steps, I made it to the bed but could not get back in. Eventually, with Nathan's help, and a few failed tries, I was in bed lying on my back again in tears. I figured something must be seriously wrong not only because the pain was getting unbearable but the way my body felt overall.

Fear was not present at all; I had to keep focused. Although there was someone else in the house with me, turning over control to him to tend to my needs did not bring me comfort; he was only eighteen years old trying to finish High School.

Another wave of pain was starting. This time, however, the pain was not the focus. Suddenly, I felt as if my energy was draining from my body, slowly from my head towards my toes.

"Nathan, hurry, call an ambulance," I said softly, even though I thought I might die before they arrived.

He did not move; instead, he offered to drive me to the hospital himself. What I did not know at the time was that he was embarrassed to have the neighbors see an ambu-

Chapter 10—The Beginning of Recovery

lance come to the house.

"No, you won't be able to get me into the car," I replied.

He left the room to make the call, and I began to pray, asking the Lord to forgive me for things I may or may not be aware of, ranging from my thoughts to deeds. It was a fast-moving prayer; I had to get everything in just in case because I thought this was it. I did not want to leave anything unaddressed as I asked the Lord to accept me.

But I did not die that morning; the ambulance came treating it as a possible heart attack, and took me to the hospital of my choice. I chose the newer hospital miles away from the one I was admitted to twice just weeks prior. Not knowing anything about doctor's hospital privileges, my choice in hospital meant none of my previous doctors would attend to me, so everyone who attended to me was all new to me and my case.

Once again, no one could pinpoint the reason for the pain, so for five more days, I was monitored and given pain medication intravenously and orally until that pain went away. It was easier for this group since I knew exactly which drug worked best.

One of the most extraordinary things from that horrible experience of feeling as if life was draining from my body was the fact that I realized I was not afraid to die. While I asked God to ease the pain, I noticed that I did not call out to Him to save my life. Instead, I focused my prayer on ensuring I would be with Him if this happened to be my time.

My will for living became a fight for defeating the sickness but not fueled out of a fear of death. I expected divine intervention from God because I had come to know that

HE IS REAL, and I had a chance to experience His power over this sickness. However, it did not take long to find out that the fight for my health was not the only battle on my hands.

Chapter 11

Easily Overlooked

Chapter 11—Easily Overlooked

My sons, Mikey and Nathan, had their individual battles with the reality of their father leaving the family and a mother's confirmed diagnosis of cancer – both within two months. More mature adults would have a hard time with that reality.

The only person they had close by was me. But my focus was on my husband's disappearance, cancer diagnosis, surgery, hospital readmissions, and pain management that I overlooked the state of mind of my sons. I never considered how they were feeling. I was able to handle myself because I knew every step to this point, but they did not. All they had was the here and now, knowing very little about its origin.
I had discussed my health with my husband in-depth but not with my children.

I dealt with our marriage from the time it was new until it was broken. I also developed a relationship with God, who was with me the entire way. I learned to trust and believe that He would never leave me. But my children - they had nothing but what they were facing at that time.

Looking back, I might have missed a few 'during work hours' events, but I was a constant support for my sons. By Mikey's sophomore year of High School and Nathan's 2nd year in Middle School, I never missed another event. It did not matter where it was or the day of the week. I had vacation time, and what a better way to use them. Ninety percent of the time, it was just me, Nathan, and a map or written directions. If it was Nathan's event, it was just me and the map. We did not have GPS back then. Mikey had track and field the first part of the year and played football towards the end of the year. The musician, Nathan, had band competitions and Football nights.

One day the boys and I were hanging out talking about the next step in their lives when I heard a change in

Mikey's voice. I looked directly at him just to see him swatting a tear from his eyes as he said, "I love you, Maw, you have been like a father and a mother to me."

"Really, why do you say that?" I asked, surprised at the statement.

He revealed some things that I did not realize that he had noticed over the years. "You don't give up – you keep trying until you cannot find another way."

On the day of surgery, they telephoned their father and pleaded with him to come back home, but he could not. One can only imagine their despair with the fear of losing their mother and being told their father would not come to be with them.

They were boys on the threshold of manhood who had never faced a crisis alone. Now they were being thrust into an adult world without warning or support.

Mikey remained calm in the crisis with his ultimate goal to make things normal again, while Nathan displayed resentment. He felt bitter about having to be the one at home left to care for me. I was the authoritative figure, so I was the parent blamed for his father's absence and whatever hate that remained over the fact that his father left him.

Nathan had noticed a wallet-sized school picture of himself on his father's nightstand. I saw the picture but thought nothing of it. But Nathan viewed it differently. It had been weeks since his father left when one afternoon, as we were talking together, he said, "He did not care enough about me to even take my picture with him." It took a second to figure out what he was saying since the statement did not fit what we were talking about. But when I realized the reason for the comment - I felt his heart. His picture was a significant sentiment that was small enough to fit in a wallet, but it

Chapter 11—Easily Overlooked

appeared to be of so little significance that it was left behind.

Nathan adored his father. I could not even imagine the pain of abandonment he was feeling to see that picture lying there and believing his father decided not to take it with him. It would become a tug of war for several years as to whom he should hate more.

He started to act up in school more than ever before. His missing school had nothing to do with taking care of me but total defiance to the rules. He would sneak out of school with his girlfriend and others who had the wheels to facilitate the behavior. Nevertheless I tried to make things as normal for him as I could. So when he asked to have a birthday 'get together' with some friends, I said yes. You could see his excitement as he clapped his fingers together a few times, swung his hand towards the other side of his body and exclaimed, "Yes! It is going down..."

By March 10th, only a few weeks after release from my third hospital stay, it was still impossible for me to move around to do anything. Nathan was glad enough that I said yes, so he had no problem taking the reins to get ready for the event. Nothing big, some music, snacks, and drinks. Knowing that things could get out of hand with no supervision, I solicited the help of Casey, a newfound friend and co-worker, the only person I knew, would not mind being a chaperone for the evening. Eighteen or not, I needed eyes watching over teenagers in my house.

Nathan would continue to struggle for the next couple of years to come as he dealt with that abandonment. I learned something about Nathan during those troublesome times. He is an extremely hard worker. It did not take long for him to accept the fact that help was limited, and he had to take care of himself. If he was passionate about something and could find a way to do it, he would surely try.

Apart from working multiple shifts at a plastic manufacturing company, he had a passion for creating musical beats, and he was very good at it. He asked to turn one of our bedrooms into a recording studio, and I allowed him to do so. He bought the equipment he needed and had that room looking the part, complete with padded walls to reduce any reflection of sound. He would spend endless hours in that room, creating music. Eventually, he connected with a group of like-minded fellows, and before long, Nathan was recording their word to his beats. This period did pass as his regular job, the ones paying his bills, demanded more of his time.

Chapter 12

The Dam is About to Burst

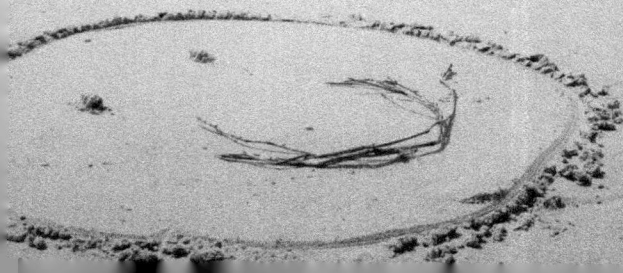

Chapter 12—The Dam Is About To Burst

There appeared a dim light at the end of my tunnel when a telephone solicitor got my attention to refinance my house. Much to my error, I divulged that I am a newly single woman with health issues and didn't think I would qualify for a refinance. Much to his remarkable find, he convinced me I would be eligible, so I entertained the possibility.

It was mid-March 2007, the real estate market had a housing bubble, and predatory lending was at its highest level. I got sucked into it. I was holding a thirteen hundred dollar a month mortgage, hospital bills, one child in high school, and the other in college; I had to do something. After all, he sounded like someone I could trust. He even gave me his cell phone number, one that supposedly only his close family had. I was encouraged to call him at any time if I had any concerns. Still not up to speed with my mobility, it took me a few days to gather the paperwork needed to apply for the refinance. I would be paying on the interest-only, causing a monthly difference of four hundred dollars per month. Joy filled my soul; I was on my way to make this thing work.

I needed a document faxed to the mortgage company by the next day, and Nathan assured me that his friend's mother could get it done at their home that evening. He was going to be in school the following day, and I could not drive myself – so why not. Several hours passed, and he did not return within the time expected, and there was no way of reaching him to find out the reason for the delay.

I was on the couch watching the television when the phone rang. As I answered it, the question came back at me, "Is this Barbara Morris?"

After confirming he was speaking to the right person, he then identified himself as a police and quickly stated the purpose of his call.

He informed me that he was with my son, who was just involved in a car accident. He also wanted to let me know that Nathan had refused an ambulance but had a friend who was on his way to take him to the hospital. He assured me that it did not appear too serious except for damage to his lip incurred from the deployed airbag from the steering wheel hitting him in the face. The car was not drivable, and I was given a telephone number to call the company where it would be towed.

The reason for the police calling me instead of my son, who was quite capable of talking, was because Nathan had informed him of his ailing mother who just had cancer surgery and multiple hospital readmissions. He had figured that if the police called me first, then it would have somehow softened the blow – it did not.

Yes, I was glad he was alive with no serious injuries, but that did not stop me from panicking. It was now late evening, but the place seemed darker than it should have. There I was, home alone, still unable to drive, and had nothing to drive to see about my child. The notion that the police might have downplayed the injuries was on my mind, and I needed to witness it for myself. My next reaction was anger for being left alone to deal with the problem.

I called his father and told him about the accident. I don't know what I presumed would happen after making the call because it was apparent that there was no degree of expectation that his father was about to go and see him.

"Have him call me," were my instructions, and they were as good as any other response I could have expected.

Casey was the only one I could think of calling. As expected, she was at my door within minutes to take me to the hospital. When we arrived, the place was full of patients

Chapter 12—The Dam Is About To Burst

– mostly little ones. A nearby children's clinic had diverted their patients to the hospital that night. So when we got to the emergency room, I found myself among a group of sick, crying children. Being in an emergency room was the last place I needed to be because getting a cold in my current condition would not be good.

Nathan was located in the middle of the chaos holding a bloody t-shirt to his face. When he is guilty of something or needs to convince someone of something, Nathan's defense mechanism is to talk excessively. This time he did not only have much to say, but he was also cursing. We have had our moments, but he was never known to use curse words in my presence before. Now his actions were totally disrespectful towards the people around him and me. He was also speaking with a high pitched voice as he fussed about having to wait since he was bleeding.

How did this all happen? Now it is evident that he had done more than the errand, and he was not giving me a clear account of earlier events.

After what seemed like an eternity, he was eventually taken to an examining room, accompanied by Casey and myself. Upon examination, it was determined that his lip was busted straight through. The force of the airbag to his face caused his teeth to cut a hole through his lip. Even though the nurse thought it was due to someone's fist. Knowing the real source of the injury, I insisted on testing for a concussion.

No damage to his brain either, so we left for home with just a few stitches to close the hole in his lip and a promise from the nurse that he will experience minimal scarring. The story I got was that the car skidded, he lost control as the vehicle swerved into the grassy median strip before it crashed into a tree.

The Cure Is In The Living

The median strip was maybe two car lengths wide, landscaped with brush and tall oak trees bearing extensively large branches separating two lanes on both sides. It is hard to figure out how he ended up hitting the tree since there is such a large spacing between all the trees in the median. It was not funny then, but that question will become a point of conversation and laughter for the years that followed.

But then I gave thanks for the tree because with the state he was in, the car would have gone straight across the median strip and ended on the other side into oncoming traffic. Right now, a few stitched and a demolished car was a blessing in comparison to the other possibility. We were blessed; Nathan was not seriously hurt, and no one else was involved in the accident.

When we got home, I called my mother with the news and asked her to take me to see about the car the following day. When we got there and saw my once new car purchased only six months before, I knew it was totaled. The area where the vehicle had collided with the tree was dead center of the front of the vehicle. The hood was dismantled, smashed windscreen, rear view mirror dangling on the sides, deployed airbag with streaks of blood and a bumper which was once attached to the front of the car was now sitting in the back seat. The gentleman who was so kind to walk me over to the now pile of metal, confirmed my observation and advised me to remove anything of value that I wanted out of it. I peered through the passenger side window in disbelief.

Have you ever seen a picture where only one item has a vibrant color, and everything else in the picture is black or grey? That was the picture stamped in my brain for weeks after visiting the wreckage. Along with the black and grey interior of my car was a single bright red solo cup laying on

Chapter 12—The Dam Is About To Burst

its side in the seat. It was evident that I had a problem on my hands. But cancer or not, I knew I had to face it since I was the only person he had.

I needed a car but did not have a vehicle to trade or down payment, but a blessing awaits. You see, when I purchased the Camry six months prior, I opted for the first time to get Guaranteed Asset Protection insurance (GAP) when it was offered; something I had declined every time I had purchased a car in the past. The GAP insurance paid off the existing car note, and I had money left over for a refund check. I was able to use that refund as a down payment for my four-year-old silver Corolla with a scar on her front cheek – it had a big scratch on the front side, but it was my car, and the monthly payment was less. But things could be worse. I refinanced the house and got a cheaper car; I knew I could make it with my salary.

April 2007, I called my job to let them know I would be returning to work within two weeks. To my shock, they had eliminated the supervisory position I had occupied before I went on sick leave. All that was available was an entry-level customer service position. It did not make sense; there appeared to be several other options, but to fight them, was not my battle; it was the Lord's. Common sense also kicked in. To look for a new job with a preexisting condition would be self-destruction. Keeping my composure, I calmly thanked her for the opportunity to continue working and hang up.

"What am I going to do?" I said to myself. Things about my situation came flooding back, including the fact that it had been four days since I completed the refinancing of my mortgage. It would have allowed me to stay in my home, but with the loss of that income, I was right back where I started.

With all that had happened for the past five months, to this point, I was not excessively sorrowful. I did not plead with anyone to change their mind, I did not mope around having pity parties, and I did not question God. But when I was told that I lost my position at the company, that was the proverbial straw that broke the camel's back – I felt like I had lost all hope of getting out of my troubles.

With my knees feeling like they were about to give way, I clutched my fingers into the deep groves on the front of my mahogany dresser to steady myself as I stared at my reflection in the mirror and released a loud cry. It was the type of scream that came from deep down in your gut; I had a lot stored there, and I just had to get the pain out. As soon as I caught my next breath, the questions came out just as loudly as I called out to my heavenly father, "God, what are you trying to tell me, what am I not doing right, what do I need to do to get from under this, why Lord, why?"

Over the months that followed, the answers to my questions were evident.

The Car: losing the expensive car and downsizing to a less costly one provided savings not only on the vehicle but gas and insurance.

The Job: He blessed me, yet again. When I returned to the job, I was placed into an accounts receivable position. It paid less than my previous salary but more than the entry-level position. I had no one to manage but myself. It was hourly pay, and I worked no more than 8 hours per day. I was able to continue healing without the stress that came with a salaried supervisory position.

Something else followed that I did not expect - church. Mid-year 2006, in a dream, I was told to resign from some of the positions I occupied at church, but I said to myself that the Pastor would not accept it without me feeling guilty of neglecting God's work, so I did not.

Now post-cancer surgery and events of the past five months, I was not strong enough to take up my church responsibilities. Due to a misunderstanding as to what I was enduring at the time, it caused a rift between myself and the administration, so I resigned and left the church.

I just wanted to heal emotionally and physically and not be judged on how fast I was doing either. That was the last 'commitment' that I had dedicated my life to that had run me into the ground. No one to supervise at work and no committees to lead at church, so now I could concentrate on just me and my children and our broken home. My new motto, if it caused you stress, remove yourself from it.

The Cure Is In The Living

Chapter 13

A New Direction

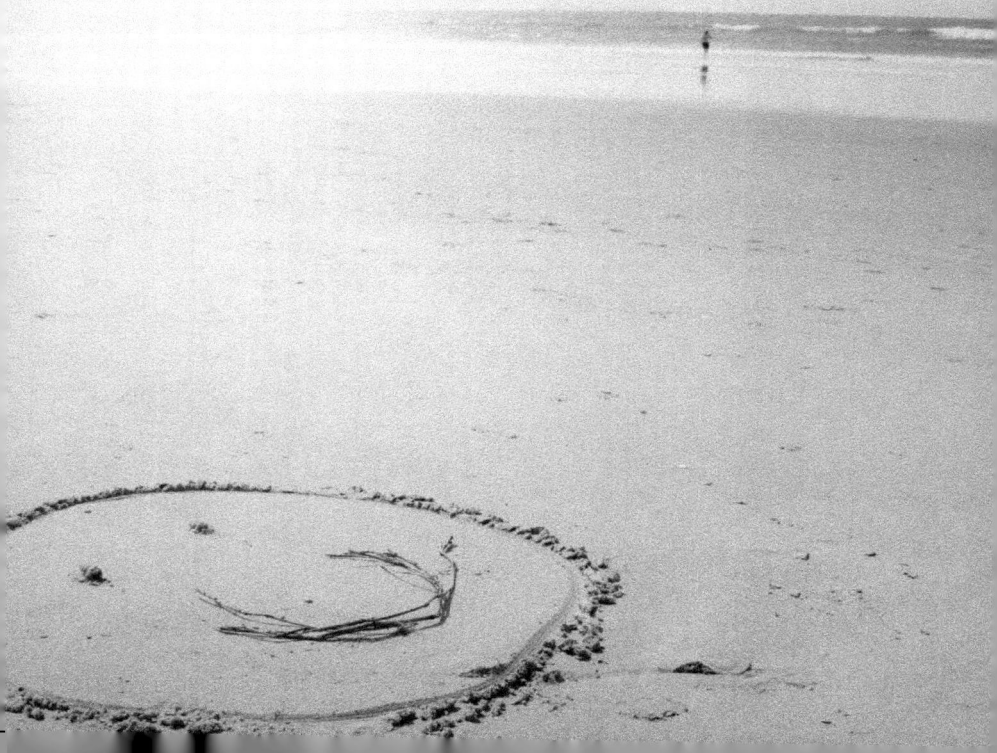

I read everything I could find regarding cancer. When I read that the survival rate is five years, I backtracked to see how many years in the past and realized how short of a time that would be. I learned that fifteen percent of cancer patients make it past five years. That was the worst bit of knowledge I could have obtained because it cast such fear and hopelessness. It was not until a friend said to me, "You will be among the 85% that survive," it was then that I started to fight to be in the higher percentage.

Since I believed that God is the source of all my needs, I marked every healing scripture I could find in my bible using strips of post-it notes with the scripture verse's location written on each piece. Each morning I read every scripture. I was so adamant about this that one morning I woke up later than usual but could still make it to work on time if I eliminated the scripture reading. On my way out the door, I turned back into the house and called the office to say I am running late. Leaving without reading those healing scriptures was not an option. One thing I knew, despite all I had lost and may lose in the future if I can keep my mind on Christ, there was a higher chance for me to make it past five years.

I also needed to change my way of thinking, and the bible verse from Ezekiel got my attention; "Rid yourselves of all the offenses you have committed, and get a new heart and a new spirit. Why will you die, people of Israel? For I take no pleasure in the death of anyone, declares the Sovereign Lord. Repent and live!" Ezekiel 18:31-32 NIV

We often do not think that the things we might have done in our past (unconfessed sins) need to be addressed. I would eventually take a few years after asking God to reveal the things I needed to confess because they did not manifest all at once. Sometimes there had to be an event that showed me why my way was not the right way.

The Cure Is In The Living

Reading the scriptures and praying at home, though, were not enough; I needed to be in a house of worship. Over the years, I had developed such an unrealistic commitment to 'church,' and not being there on a Sunday morning was earth-shattering. Why so dramatic? Well, attending all church activities had become the norm for me. The word in the church was that only what you do for Christ will last. On Sundays, I attended morning and evening service and was also required to preach two Sundays a month. Then I would return for Bible study each Tuesday night and prayer meeting on Thursday nights.

But that was not all. Other positions were assigned to me by leadership because they trusted my ability to carry out the duties. My other responsibilities at church included serving as secretary for the church and finance committee, choir leader, and event planner - just to name a few. Ironically, I was not doing it unto the Lord; I was just working for the church – the institution.

One morning while I was praying, I heard that whisper in my spirit, "Genesis 12." I grabbed my bible and turned to the book of Genesis, chapter 12, and started to read from verse one. I did not make it past verse 5 because I could no longer see the words on the page clearly through the tears.

"The Lord had said to Abram, "Go from your country, your people and your father's household to the land I will show you. I will make you into a great nation, and I will bless you; I will make your name great, and you will be a blessing. I will bless those who bless you, and whoever curses you I will curse; and all peoples on earth will be blessed through you." So Abram went, as the Lord had told him; and Lot went with him. Abram was seventy-five years old when he set out from Harran. 5 He took his wife Sarai,

Chapter 13—A New Direction

his nephew Lot, all the possessions they had accumulated and the people they had acquired in Harran, and they set out for the land of Canaan, and they arrived there. Gen 12:1-5 NIV

I believed this was confirmation that my time at my current church was over. But it brought a question; where is Mount Canaan for me? I felt lost without a place of worship because it was customary for me to be in church on Sundays. For several weeks I did not get an answer as to where the Lord wanted me to worship. I did not want to be in a church if I could not praise Him freely, so I went searching for Pentecostal churches in the telephone directory and did not find one that felt right. One day I heard in my spirit "Baptist." Since I don't know of Baptist churches clapping hands and shaking a tambourine, I was in disbelief and thought I had not heard correctly.

That was until the night my friend Debbie called. "I am checking on you, sis," she said with her cheerful self.

I told her I was struggling a bit, but ok. You know the way we do. We are feeling lousy, doubtful, but because we are believers, to show spiritual strength, we still say we are ok, and God is good – but honestly not quite feeling it. Trying to divert the attention away from me, I inquired about her, but she stopped me mid-sentence and said, "you know what, you need to get out of the house. Meet me downtown tomorrow evening for dinner – my treat. I will not take no for an answer." Reluctantly, I accepted. She stated that she would not take no for an answer. And well, I could not come up with a lie that would sound believable.

Tomorrow came quicker than I would have liked. We sat together at one table while her husband and daughters were seated at a few tables back from us. I learned then that Friday was their family night, but she knew she needed to

The Cure Is In The Living

spend some time with her friend. As if she knew the source of my condition, the first conversation question she asked was, "So how is Church?" This question I answered honestly and shared my current dilemma. One thing about my friend, she never seemed to allow the person talking to finish their thought before she interjected her opinion, and this time was no different.

Again, halfway through my story, she interrupted, so I shoved a forkful of food in my mouth as I waited for her point of view. "Well, I don't know if you would be interested, but you can come worship with us at Mount Cannan."

Immediately I remembered the scripture Genesis 12 – when God told Abram to leave his kindred and that they left and went forth into the land of Canaan. I dropped my fork and reached for my napkin to cover my mouth that was now full of food, and asked, "What did you just say?" taking a swallow, and I continued, "What is the name of your church?' "Mount Canaan," she replied. "Do they openly praise God? I mean… Are they not afraid to raise or clap their hands in worship?" I asked anxiously.

"Yes, it's a missionary Baptist Church."

"It's a Baptist Church?" I said in disbelief – is this happening right now?

"Yes, it is. Why?" she replied, now puzzled regarding my odd behavior and sudden transformation from gloom to joy.

I shared with her my "Baptist" and "Genesis 12" revelation. I was able to get to the end this time without interruptions, and as I concluded, I said with a light-hearted broad smile, "I will be there on Sunday. What time does the church service begin?"

Chapter 13—A New Direction

We finished our meal with a joyous feeling believing that I am going to be just fine. Everything else of importance that I had seemed to have lost was starting to come back, and that was an excellent feeling. I did not doubt that Mt. Canaan Missionary Baptist Church was going to be my new church home even though I have never been in the building or heard the pastor preach. I praised God in my car all the way home. I did hear correctly, and I knew I was following His leading. The songwriter sings, "there is a balm in Gilead to soothe the sin-sick soul" Mt. Canaan became my Gilead for five years. They were there for times when I was short on food or even that cold winter when the central heat in my house was not working, and I was so cold, my fingers would be numb.

I accept that the falling out with the church I was previously was also a part of God's plan. After all, I was afraid of resigning when he told me to, even when I knew it was too much. Wow! I actually found joy in all my afflictions when I could see them as blessings.

My life changed. Throughout the year, I had scheduled CT scans to make sure that the cancer had not returned. First, it was every three months, and by the time it got to six months, I was not as anxious about the results. But boy was I glad when they told me everything was clear. It had become a formality. The changes also applied to my eating habits when I eliminated red meat, processed food, and junk food. I replaced those with a balanced diet, and most importantly, NO SUGAR in any form.

I walked every morning even if it was still dark outside at 6:00 a.m. and again in the evening after work. I made sure I went outside for my lunch breaks and took a half-hour nap in my car most of the time. My weight loss of 26 pounds was misunderstood by many as being due to having cancer, but nothing was further from the truth. I was happier now and no longer overworked. I was able to reduce my stress. I looked and felt healthier than I had been for years and was able to keep it that way for the next eight (8) years with regular CT scans, which had now moved to once per year.

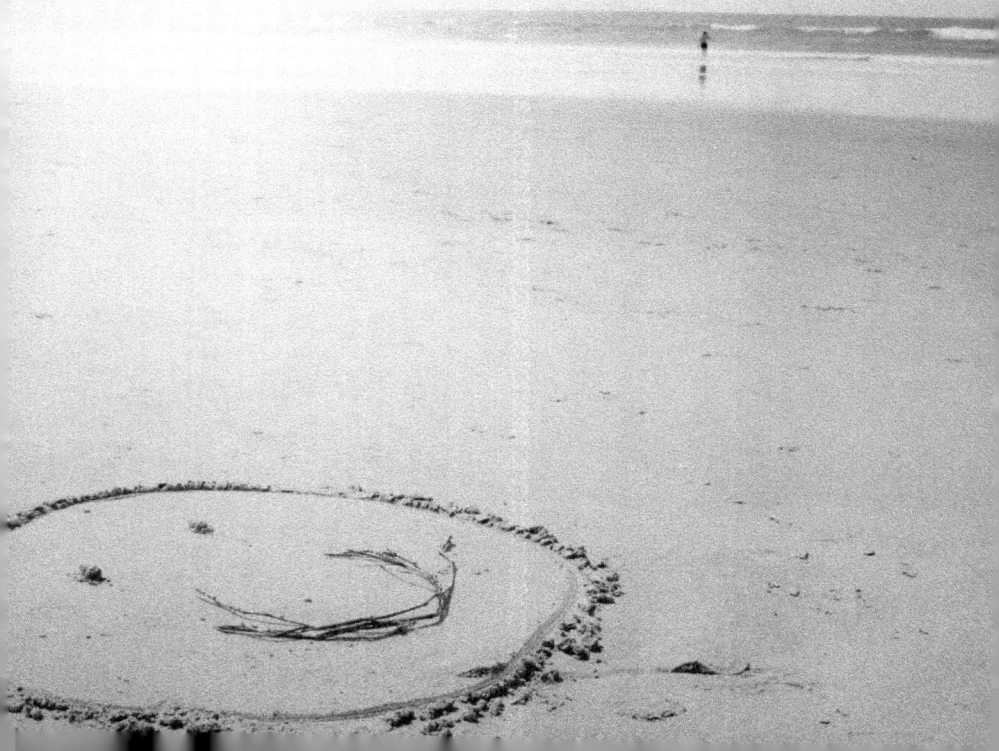

Chapter 14

It's Back

By the beginning of my 9th year of being cancer-free, I had been living in Tampa for four years. Tampa is where the love of my life had returned. No, it was not a man, even though that would not be a bad idea. No, it was working stressful hours and my love for sugar-sweets, or whatever we want to call it. Ice cream, chocolate, cakes, pies were my greatest weakness. Although none of them ever made the grocery list, they would somehow be in my grocery cart at checkout. I would make an ice cream run to the gas station for a pint of Ben & Jerry's chocolate fudge brownie ice cream like someone who runs out to get a six-pack. If I craved it, I had to have it, and it would all be eaten in one sitting.

The second love of my life also came back – my love of pleasing others through hard work and long hours. I had to keep my deadlines, and woe to me if I allowed my boss to think I was not good at my job.

Approaching the end of my 10th year (in 2016), I had a dream. I saw a snake a distance away, and although I usually am afraid, I was not worried because it was so far away from me. In a flash, the snake sprang from where it was towards me and consumed ¾ of my left hand. I woke up with the thought – I am in trouble again. What was I to do? I could not change the dream, and I did not know what type of trouble to prevent, so that is all it was – just an inconclusive interpretation of a dream.

By August, I was having headaches, and my blood pressure would not regulate even though I was on medication. My friend Sonia insisted that I go to the emergency room. I did not want to go, so I told her I would watch it and see. As the days turned into weeks without change, I figured I probably should get this checked out, so I took my shower, washed my hair, did my blow and hot curl, and packed an overnight bag – just in case.

The Cure Is In The Living

Minutes after one in the afternoon of Saturday, August 13th, I was tossing that overnight bag onto the front passenger seat as I headed to the emergency room. That is how you operate when you live alone. Advanced planning minimizes the need to call on others for help. I had enough in that bag to last me a week at the hospital.

As I backed out of the parking space, I heard that soft voice, "This is how it happened the first time you had a cancer diagnosis – you drove to the emergency room by yourself for a non-related issue." I took a deep breath and voiced a short prayer asking the Lord to stay with me through the process. It had been about six months since my last scan, but whatever the outcome, I had to be brave – no time to panic.

When I got to triage in the emergency room, and they took my blood pressure reading, it was so high they rushed me into a room immediately. Multiple teams were working at the same time. There were EKG machines, scanners, and x-ray machines that were brought to the room as they frantically tried to figure out the reason for my severely elevated blood pressure reading. I had so many questions being thrown at me. I just had to stop speaking for a bit. Noticing that my anxiety level was rising, someone in the room apologized, "So sorry, but when we have someone with such a high blood pressure reading, we must work quickly to try and figure out why." At the end of all the tests and imaging results, doctors detected a new spot on my lung. The cancer was back. I was not frightened – I felt no different than before I heard the words, but I knew it was time to call someone, and my son Mikey got the first call.

By October 21, 2016, I had a left thoracotomy with wedge resection of the left lower lobe mass, reportedly a stage IA lung cancer. At 57 years of age, I never felt nor

Chapter 14—It's Back

looked old. I never complained about birthdays but celebrated that I was able to see another one. This time only 50 days from my 58th birthday, I looked and felt beaten and worn out. Suddenly it had become difficult to cope emotionally during the months that followed. The fact that I was cancer-free again due to surgery did not bring my spark back.

According to my surgeon, because it had been ten years since the first cancer diagnosis, the likelihood was exceptionally high that this was new cancer that happens to be in my lung - like the first. This posed the question: "will I be able to do it again and keep this parasite out of my body?" My answer was, all I needed to do was go back to my healthy lifestyle.

My physical health was not the only thing that had become somewhat unstable. Spiritually, I was losing my connection with my church, although my faith in God remained constant. I was extremely thankful to God for the early detection, for safe surgery, for clean margins, and, most of all, I was alive.

Emotionally, however, I felt let down when, for two months, I was out of church but had not heard from a few key people who I considered friends. This took me back to times where people would use me to do for them, but that was as far as it went. Pretentious friendships were revealed, so naturally, I did not feel at home anymore when I returned. When someone thinks of themselves as a part of something – like a family, and then when trials come, and they do not feel supported by that family, it hurts. Justifiably or not, the struggle is real.

The church was also changing, and the requirements for leadership members had increased. One of those changes was the requirement that any leadership member was expected to be at church at 7:30 am to meet before Sunday school. Sunday school would then be followed by Sunday morning worship and any other departmental meeting that might happen.

It wasn't long after that I noticed that I was feeling good and ready to go each Sunday morning when I got up. However, by the time I got dressed and about to leave the apartment, I would start feeling weak or short of breath - even to the point of wheezing. Sometimes I forced myself to go, but it would keep happening repeatedly. It got so bad that I was having heart palpitations as diagnosed by a doctor. One of the Pastors whom I believed to be a friend suggested that my condition was *psychological.* You have come to the same conclusion – haven't you?

One of the ministries I was still involved in was the Prayer ministry. But with one foot in and one foot out, my interest dwindled. We would meet once per week after Sunday morning service, and to fill the time, spoke about some issues at hand, prayed, and went home. I felt we needed more. So when the Pastor asked me to assist with the prayer ministry as co-coordinator, I said yes. I was excited about the prospect of being a part of the leadership of this ministry. My desire was for spiritual growth within the department, to be able to share ideas that could hopefully build onto what we already had. Especially since they had taken on being physically present in the church and openly beseeching prayer requests.

The Coordinator and I had planning meetings with the head of Ministries as we shared ideas of prayer retreats and guidance as to how best to approach others needing prayer. In other words, things to strengthen those prayer warriors who would be standing on the spiritual battlefield. But while the ideas were accepted and the excitement was high,

Chapter 14—It's Back

the tentative dates would change or simply fall off the schedule. In my view, we were still in the same place, with no sign of improvement. By no means do I hold anyone at fault. Instead, I surmised that my perception of what was needed was not the same as those who could make the change.

Anxiety and disappointments still did not mean I needed to leave the church – nope, God did not tell me to go. That was my story, and I was sticking to it.

My friend Melvin, who was newly diagnosed with stage 4 cancer, was in a similar state of mind. He badly wanted to preach the word of God – in his own voice. But again, it was made clear that his voice did not meet the standards of that church. He would get excited and leap two steps forward to only find himself tossed even further back when told his way was incorrect.

Discouraged, he decided he would just sit back and not preach again until the day he found someone who would mentor and foster the calling he knew he had, which was to be a preacher. True to the form of a true friend, he called me. "Barbara, I found us a church," he said to me. And my reply, "Us? I don't know about that. God did not release me from the church I was currently attending and I am not going anywhere until then." I wished him and his family well and shared in his excitement that he finally found someone who understood him and was willing to allow him to be himself and still preach the word.

By the time I recovered from one of my anxieties one Sunday morning in August, it was late, so I decided I would visit Melvin and his family at their new place of worship.

As I took a seat towards the back of the church, I could identify a familiar song being played by a gentleman on the keyboard. Others were greeting and talking with each other as I frantically scanned the area looking for the familiar faces of my friends. They were not present, but I figured they would show up in a few. As I looked around the remainder of the sanctuary, the thought came to me – why are you here; what purpose would be served from a change of plans causing you to be here this morning. I am a firm believer that things do not happen by chance. So I asked, "Lord, why am I here?" I would like to believe that the answer came back immediately, "could it be my husband is here."

Just then, the music stopped. I looked up to see the gentleman who was playing the keyboard stepped down from the platform, which represented the altar. He had made only a few steps when I looked outside to see if my friends came in as it appears that church service is about to begin. No such luck, so I went back to my thoughts, which brought more questions than anything else. To have an idea about a husband was funny to me since I had come to terms with my singleness. Outside of that, I had developed a fear of getting involved with someone again just to find out it was a mistake after marriage. At fifty-seven, that would be devastating, so I was quite content with my status in life. So most naturally, I chuckled inside and was about to dismiss the thought when that same internal voice chimed up again, "No, don't dismiss the thought – remember the details just in case it does happen."

I looked up again across the sanctuary, and the man who was playing the keyboard was now halfway down the hallway, where he was speaking and laughing with the person operating the soundboard. This time I noticed him, he appeared to be slightly below average height, very slender, dark-skinned, very casually dressed, did I say very…a few times…I meant all of them. I thought nothing more of him as I looked in the opposite direction, thinking, "Well, he is not my type, so that is not him."

Chapter 14—It's Back

The service started, and everyone was in their respective places. It became apparent that the person who was on the keyboard when I walked in was not the designated keyboard player but the drummer. As he took his place behind the drums, the real keyboard player entered, followed by the guitarist. I pulled out my phone and discreetly as I could, text Melvin asking if he will be attending church service that morning. His response was, "No – I am at a bowling tournament today, but I will be there next week."

Three young ladies entered the platform - It was time for praise and worship. Well, I am already here, let's do this – no more idle thoughts. When church service was over, I figured I would sneak out since my purpose for going was not to find a church for myself. My mission was to evaluate the church for my friend, and my task was done.

My report was that the teaching and preaching were excellent, which opened a door for him once again to say, "We found ourselves a new church, and you should come over and join with my family. "Although it had been a short time, they were pleased there. I rebuked him again, saying, "God did not tell me to leave my church to come over there with you all."

Several weeks passed as I continued with my Sunday morning anxiety and my friend's nudging that I am responsible for my peace of mind and how much of an asset I would be over there. "Why don't you call the pastor and talk with him?" he asked, getting tired of me saying no. I figured what would it hurt to speak with Pastor Neely, so I scheduled a telephone meeting but later canceled the phone call. The closer the date came, the more pressed I felt to meet in person, so I changed the appointment to a face-to-face meeting.

As I sat on the red couch of Pastor Neely's office, he asked what I did at my current church. I was in an entrance interview without knowing it. I was forthcoming with my feelings of being a licensed minister, but my present church did not provide a license to ministers who joined their church. We talked of some of the other things I had been doing, but what got his attention was my prayer ministry involvement. The position of leader of the prayer ministry was currently vacant at the Mill.

At the end of the meeting, I thanked him for his time, but my mind had not changed. I had no intention of leaving my current place of worship. There would be a meeting with the ministers at my church, and I was hoping I would get some encouragement to move forward. I never made the meeting.

It was a Tuesday evening in September 2017. On my way to the meeting, my son called, asking if I had prepared for the storm. Shocked, I wondered what storm. "Ma, are you telling me you have not done or bought anything to prepare for the storm – for real?"

"No," I replied, "I don't know what you are talking about, seriously."

"Mom, you cannot find a bottle of water in a Wal-Mart store up here – they are all sold out. I just came back from Tampa, where my company sent me to pick up a load of bottled water to bring back to Ocala."

That explained all the long lines I noticed at several gas stations along the way. I reassured him that I would stop by the supermarket and get some stuff. I had a choice, ministers meeting or storm preparation. Within a few minutes, I pulled into the parking lot of the next supermarket. The parking lot of Publix was full, and on the inside, the shelves were bare. No bread, canned foods, or water on the shelves. Now, when even the expensive 'healthy' loaves of bread are gone,

Chapter 14—It's Back

you know you have a problem. That's how I learned of the oncoming hurricane, Irma. I don't know how I missed the warnings, but I did.

Once again, I thought that I had failed by not attending the minister's meeting, and I was not going to be looked upon very well due to my absence. I weighed guilt against, possibly being unprepared for a category five storm, and the fear of the storm won.

On September 10, 2017, Irma went across the State of Florida as a category four hurricane. I waited out the storm with my sons and their family that weekend, and by the beginning of the following week, the Lord had released me from my home church. That familiar still voice in my spirit was clear that the Lord was sending me there not for what I can get from that church but sharing with them what he had already given me. By now, I had been cancer-free for eleven months, and my next scan was scheduled for mid-December.

The exit interview was on September 14, 2017. I felt I would sound silly and would be judged if I tried to explain that I decided to leave based on several consecutive dreams. Even though I had learned over the years that that is the way the Lord gives me directions, I was very cautious with whom I shared that information. What others thought of me was still an issue at this point—another weakness I needed to put under subjection.

And so, I shared only part of my reason as I explained my weekly anxieties and the fact that I felt guilty for not fulfilling the requirements of my position. As leaders, the members expected and almost required our presence at weekly bible studies, early Sunday morning huddles, business meetings, etc. It was actually not an unreasonable request. But for me, I felt and stressed that if I could not live by the rules as mandated, I needed to get out, and that was what I was about to do. I resigned. Pastor Way had one question for me, which was, "Have you found a church home." And without hesitation, I answered "yes," but I had not started full attendance there as yet.

As we left, I felt an odd feeling of leaving something special – but no doubts. As Pastor Way had mentioned, I had participated in the church in several capacities and had made some close relationships. I don't do well with cutting loose without making sure everyone is ok – as if anyone would care about me being concerned.

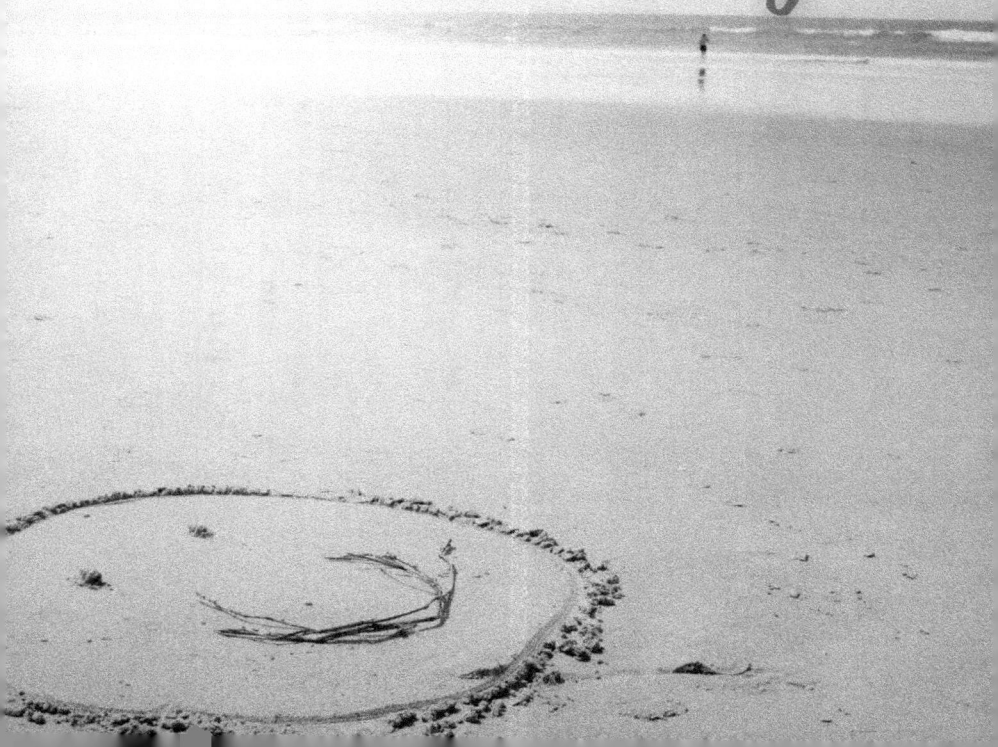

Chapter 15

A New Journey

My third visit to The Mill ended up being my acceptance of membership. I dressed differently than most because I was accustomed to do so. It did not take long, though, to realize it was a come as you are congregation. To my surprise, this same laid-back approach was what gave me comfort for years to come. At The Mill, I felt I was not judged and less scrutinized. I did not wonder if I was dressed well enough or if I am being laughed at because my shoes were not fashionable. I did not feel inferior but felt at home. Here I felt confident that I had something to give. And most of all, a ministerial license was within my grasp – at least that was what I thought.

I became the Director of the Prayer ministry immediately, but first things first, I needed Prayer Ministry members.

The idea of creating a class to teach the congregation the effective ways of praying was on the table. It was a simple task if you just wanted to say you taught a class on praying – it's another to grasp the vision and have something that will impact the participant.

Does that mean it's not possible to create a class on praying that would hold an audience? Of course not. But we first need them to get there. I continued working and pulling materials to conjure up a class on how to pray. A deadline was given and passed with lots of content to present.

December 1, 2017, general results from another 6-month follow-up reads: "Most recent results - Patient notified that her recent CT is stable. Routine post op changes are seen, no adenopathy, effusions and no evidence of recurrence. She is otherwise doing well and I will reschedule her next appointment out 6 months with CT on the day of her visit as we discussed." Once again, I was eternally thankful for the good results – no evidence of recurrence - are fantastic words.

The Cure Is In The Living

I woke up earlier than necessary on December 3rd thinking I needed to get to church at 7:30a.m., when I suddenly remembered that I had changed churches. No matter how hard I tried, I just could not fall back to sleep, so I got up and proceeded with my usual Sunday morning preparation. The Mill had changed to two services recently, one at 8:30 a.m. and the other at 11:00 a.m. each Sunday; I chose the 11 a.m. to be my time for worship. But to my surprise this morning, no matter how slow I moved around, I was fully dressed and ready to go way before even the first service would begin. So I sat down for a while to wait it out when the thought occurred why wait it out here, just go on to church – no harm in being in both services.

I arrived a few minutes before 8:00a.m. to find the drummer; you may remember him to be the 'not my type' guy, standing by the door looking puzzled. Pastor Neely was the only other person there also looking perplexed standing by his open car door with cell phone in hand.

As I approached the two gentlemen, Pastor blurted that Tony forgot to set up. I looked at the drummer and said, "oh, boy." The issue with this situation is that the Mill uses fresh bread and not wafers for communion, so no bread – no element – no communion.

Without being asked, I went into my 'solution' mode, no use standing around "One of us can drive to the nearby supermarket to get the bread and the other two can get the vessels cleaned and pour the wine." I figured that we had enough time to get everything done if we hurry, but the worst-case scenario would be that we serve the sacraments later than we usually do.

"Sure, yes, yes – that will work. I will go to the store, and you guys can start setting up." Pastor jumped into his

Chapter 15—A New Journey

Chrysler, and the drummer and I hustled to the kitchen with me at his mercy. I had no idea where to find anything nor what their set-up entails. I had only experienced two communions there, and I had not paid much attention to it in the past.

The first time I witnessed communion here, it was different than what I was accustomed to seeing. Real bread pinched into bite-sized pieces was used instead of wafers, grape juice in the familiar tiny cups for the congregation, but wine for the ministers at the communion table served in crystal stem glasses. There had to be a good size piece of bread on the table used to demonstrate the breaking of the bread.

By the second time, I was distracted by the struggle with taking off the plastic wrap that was securing the freshness of the pinched bits of bread on the tray. My next concern was the nearby long stem glasses with wine. One wrong pull of that plastic wrap and there would definitely be a spill. I could see the frustration on Pastor's face, and smiled on the inside. My inappropriate amusement was not at his frustration but as to why the plastic wrap was still covering the tray. I spent the rest of the communion experience focusing on how I could fix what I now viewed as "a problem."

"Where are the communion trays and cups? Where is the grape juice?" I started asking questions as if I was left in charge. I quickly realized that it was a 'seek and find' also for the drummer as we tried to figure it out - quickly.

Within minutes we had the bread trays washed and ready for the arrival of the bread. The trademark plastic cups were placed in the communion tray, and the drummer was gingerly pouring grape juice in them as he instructed me to pour a few sips of wine in the eight-ounce stemware for the communion table. The bread came, and I went into cutting half of it into bite size pieces.

The Cure Is In The Living

No, pinching would not work for me – it was too far from being out of uniform. We made it on time; the communion table was set and ready for the first service. Now this time I paid attention to everything that was being done at that communion table. I wanted to see if I messed up.

By the time the first service was over, the drummer and I were a team - experts, if you will. As we removed the unused elements to set up for the next service, I had some time to reflect on exactly how the Pastor's hands moved over the table – so to speak. I stood there for a second, staring at the table and going over in my head how to rearrange it to make it easier for the server.

Now let's be clear, this had nothing to do with Pastor's ability to perform communion flawlessly; after all, he had been doing this format for years – way before me and my opinions came onboard. The problem was me. Remember Murphy's Law... Anything that can go wrong, will go wrong. For me that means, because it can go wrong, if I see the problem, I need to do what I can to decrease the chance that something will go wrong.

This is how I see that slim chance of a disaster. It would be the one time where the plastic wrap gives way as he tugs at it causing his cufflinks to hit the glass of wine between him and the now exposed bread...I won't have to add anything new to prove my point. Remember the reason I was pulled into this in the first place is because someone forgot to set up communion? That someone was Deacon Tony, who had been setting up communion for years and not once did he forget a communion Sunday and miss setting up – until now. Was it a problem or a purpose? You will be the judge.

Not realizing I was being watched as I stood staring at the table, I heard the drummer, "what are you thinking?"

Chapter 15—A New Journey

Surprised, I looked up and smiled, "How did you know I was thinking about something?"

"I could tell," he responded without missing a beat. "I don't like the flow; it's not realistic. With Pastor stretching over glasses with wine to get to the sacrament trays, it's an accident waiting to happen."

We both walked back to the kitchen and completed preparation for the next service. As I cut the bread in my one size for all cubes, a bit of the extremely hard crust fell into the plate. I was standing by the counter in my own world and a silly thought popped into my head which in turn prompted a snicker loud enough that the drummer heard it.

The drummer, now apparently watching every move I made asked "What are you laughing at?" "Oh, nothing really, a piece of the hard crust was mingled into the bread and I was just saying to myself that I better get it out — wouldn't want anyone to break their dentures on it."

He started laughing, although I did not think it warranted such a robust laugh then said "mmm, you got jokes." In his Trinidadian accent he continued, "I am a very observant person and I notice since you have been here that you have a magnificent mind." That was the first personal compliment I received from the drummer.

Most people would simply say thank you, but that is not what happened here. You see, that magnificent mind he mentioned is always wondering why, how and what — so I noticed the tone, the look, and the smile that accompanied the statement. Adamant that I did not want to encourage anything, I said "Believe me, you don't want to observe this mind of mine. It comes up with some crazy stuff sometimes." We both laughed as I picked up the bread plate and started for the sanctuary.

Still not sure if I would be overstepping my bounds, I asked "Is there a reason why you guys have the sacraments placed in this fashion?" "No, you can change it if you want." And so I did. It was the beginning of a new layout to how the communion table would be set up for future Sundays. I found the gold-plated covers for each bread service and replaced the 8-ounce stemware with short 2-ounce liqueur glasses. Instead of pouring the wine in the glasses ahead of time, I got a glass salad dressing decanter to serve as a wine decanter. All symmetrically proportioned with the other vessels. Now he could break the bread and pour the wine just before service at the table.

Redoing the communion table was not the only good that came out of Deacon forgetting that it was First Sunday. That faithful first Sunday broke the ice for the drummer and the Minister.

I had my scan in December 2017 with no concerns because I was banking on multiple years of being cancer free as I did previously, so I was very happy with the clear results. December proved to be an excellent month for me that year; I was also blessed to witness the marriage of Nathan to Ashley, his high school sweetheart.

As weeks went by, the drummer and I found ourselves having lengthy conversations and debates. In one incident, in particular, we were talking about places we would like to travel, which led into a biblical discussion with a Q and A exchange that lasted almost 8 hours. We earned more than anyone could monetarily pay us for 8 hours – the time was exciting and priceless. We tested each other's religious beliefs and our understanding of certain passages in the bible. I avoided most of the personal questions about myself as I had learned not to tell a man the things you like because,

Chapter 15—A New Journey

more than likely, his actions towards you will reflect what you are expecting instead of who he really is. So, I played my cards very close to the chest. As we conversed, I found out that we had insanely similar interests. The places we wish to travel, how we viewed a Christian home should be, foods we do not like - just to name a few. However, the greatest excitement came with our discussion of God's word. There were times that we disagreed, but boy did it cause each of us to extend our thinking and research for a greater understanding of the word. It was refreshing, stimulation and fun all rolled up in one.

It did not take the drummer long to know what he wanted – he viewed this as an answer to his prayers. A month into our 'serious' friendship, he told me how he felt and that we were going to get married, and there is no turning back. I said a quick prayer "Please, Lord don't let him ask me if I felt the same way." I did not want to hurt his feelings by saying no. Don't judge me now; after all, it had only been three weeks for me. My response was an attempt to put the brakes on this fast moving love train.

"Are you that sure?" Followed with, "To take me as your wife would be taking someone with serious health issues. Although I have been blessed and am a cancer survivor, you do realize…"

The drummer did not allow me to finish before his rebuttal. "The love between us is not based solely on the physical but more on the spiritual – God created this. From the first day you visited the church, and I saw you sitting there, I said to myself - that is wife potential. I did not know I would ever see you again. You were seated and all I saw was your face and upper body – this was not derived from lust. Since you joined the church, I have been watching you all these months. I see how you relate to others and how they relate to you. I have been impressed by the sermons you preached. I am serious and you can start designing your ring – there is no turning back."

What was there for a sister to say but "ok" in a questionable tone.

As Pastor so eloquently voiced it in later months; *who would believe that the screw-up of a Deacon would spark the union of the drummer and the Minister.*

Chapter 16

There is Definitely Going to be a Wedding

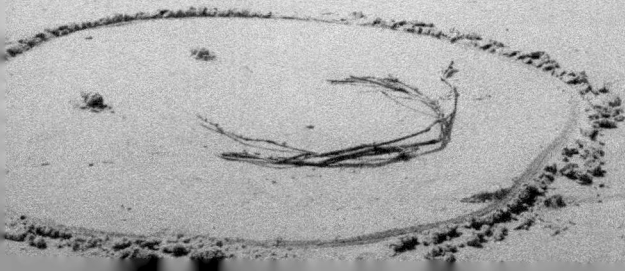

Surprisingly enough, I was not fighting what the drummer had to say. I was not against remarrying – but I was so mindful that I did not want to do anything to influence and draw the wrong person. I needed to be sure whoever came was sent by God and not selected by me. I looked at what I wanted (the physical view) versus what God had been saying about the situation (the spiritual view), and even though I 'thought' I was missing some of my requests in the physical viewpoint, I knew deep within me – the spiritual was on point. If I allowed this to pass by because he didn't meet all of my requirements, I would have missed God's gift for me for the rest of my life. So this was when my prayer changed from "what I wanted in a husband" to "give me the heart to receive your gifts as you see fit for me – and also prepare me to take care of that gift whereby we would both be blessed for being obedient to your will for our lives." When I was able to view my situation through the eyes of God, I realized that I too had a responsibility for the gift God was about to give me. It was not only for me to have someone to care for me.

Well, the man said no turning back – so I focused on moving forward in planning our lives together. But I was being bothered by the fact that I did not feel afraid or anxious. Me, the person who questions everything to death, was not asking if I was making a mistake, or am I moving too fast, or the dreaded, "What will others think?" I was A-ok. One morning as I was praying, I asked the Lord why am I not scared. Immediately I heard the words "perfect love casteth out fears," which is a part of 1 John 4:18. It was after then that I allowed myself to accept what was before me. Somewhere along the way, I had also fallen in love with the drummer without realizing it. What an awesome God we serve. He takes care of us even when we are not thinking about it.

About two weeks later, I was in the mall and passed a

jewelry store advertising custom-made service, so I stopped in to grab the information to share on our phone call later. Just like the speed of everything else in my life for the past couple of months, the upcoming annual event was only three days away. The jewelers will be coming into the store for one-on-one sessions with customers desiring special pieces and services. When the attendant asked if I would like to schedule a time to speak with the jeweler, I was sure she would not have a time that would work for the drummer since he lived and worked over two hours away on a low traffic day. But, sure enough, they had the perfect appointment time slot still opened to facilitate the drummer's travel time. They proceeded with their mini interview to get an idea of what type of ring I was looking for, so I explained the perfect ring.

Oh, let me back up for a bit. What is the perfect ring? Yep – there is a story there as well.

It is now January 2018, but over 15 years ago, I dreamed that I was getting married to a man who loved me – I could actually feel the love being extended. I remember he was willing to make a personal sacrifice to be with me because he was certain that our love was true. The odd thing was his eyes were as blue as an aquamarine gemstone. At the time of the dream, I was married to my first husband – so I dismissed it. Years later, after I was divorced, the memory of the dream came up, and I said, if I ever get married again, I will find a way to put that blue stone in my engagement ring even though it might not be popular.

So a week before I went to the mall, I was reminded again about the blue stone. As I got to the corner of Congress Ave and Ridge Road in New Port Richey, I said aloud. "Lord, what is the significance of the aquamarine stone?" The whole thing unfolded as I waited for the traffic light to change back to green. The answer was, Aqua is water – water always takes the shape of its container. In the same manner, no matter the shape your lives should take, your love for each other will conform to it. And Marine is the sea – ocean to depict the depth of our love.

Now standing in the store before the salesperson, sure enough, she asked why an aquamarine stone instead of a diamond. As I shared my dream and explanation, it touched her, she proceeded to share my romantic sentiment with everyone in the store.

We kept our appointment and met with the custom jeweler, who brought a few rings that matched my earlier description of what I wanted. We agreed on one that gave even more meaning to our pending union. It had three bands that spread out halfway from the side up to the center, to support the main setting which was a two-tier pear shape setting of diamonds; with a pear-shaped aquamarine center stone. What added to it being perfect was that the pear shapes looked like the shape of drops of water. It was my size – a perfect fit, and it didn't need anything except for my aquamarine stone to be set and polished. We left the store with the ring that same night.

No, we did not forget the drummer's ring. He got measured and selected the ring he wanted. He was not as lucky, though – they did not have his size in the store. My ring finger was a perfect size 7, and he was a perfect size 11. The 7/11 ring sizes created a little excitement among the three ladies that were now attending to us, relating it to the once-popular '7-Eleven' convenience stores.

There had been so many similarities and nuances between us that we started to find them funny. For example, just to name a few, we both owned a Toyota Camry manufactured in the same year, and they were the same color – Predawn Grey. I had the Sports Edition, and he had the Luxury Edition (I call it the Laidback edition), and they depicted our personality quite well. The drummer's license plate was a sign of love for me. My interpretation, '100% for Barbara and Roger.' How cute is that? Ok, maybe not?

Yes, the drummer's name is Roger, and we were married five months later at a small June wedding. This time I had my June wedding simply because other dates would clash with my busy work schedule, and waiting a year at our age was just downright stupid. After all, neither of us were millionaires, so we were not marrying for money, and the possibility of pregnancy being the reason would have been the greatest stupidity of all. We were just two mature people who wholeheartedly believed that God brought us together and gave us a second chance at love.

June was a busy month between the wedding and work. My next six month CT scan was also due. Since I went ten years from the first cancer surgery to the time it occurred again. I had a comfort level that the cancer was not coming back any time soon, if at all; I should make it beyond ten years this time if I go back to eating healthy. With that confidence, I rescheduled the June appointment for July because it presented a conflict with our honeymoon.

The honeymoon was a five-night Caribbean cruise to the Bahamas. It was my third cruise and Roger's first, so I had an idea of things to expect. For example, at the onset of purchasing a cruise the question, "Is this a special occasion," usually leaves you with an assumption that a surprise awaits you on board. That would be exciting for most people, but to an extreme introvert, that can be toxic. A case in point was our first night in the formal dining room. As we took our seats, I could see the disgust on Roger's face as the dining room staff danced around a table singing happy birthday to someone seated across the room. I could see their embarrassment on Roger's face, so you can imagine what happened when it was our turn – I knew it was coming, but he did not. It is not for me to spoil a surprise, though, so we ordered our meal and were halfway through when it happened.

That was my first lesson on Roger's way of showing his displeasure at something someone had done. In a quick motion, he pulled his chin towards his chest just enough to be able to look over the top of his wireframe glasses with a questionably wide-eyed piercing steer. That was the look I got as the voice over the intercom prompted everyone to applaud for the newlywed: Barbara and Roger Thomas, who had joined the voyage for their honeymoon.

There we were dressed for a night on the town – well ship in this case. Me in my knee-length dress with its close-fitting bodice attached to a flowing skirt with six-inch pleats. The satin reflective fabric had a floral print of deep ruby and burgundy colored roses accompanied by deep green leaves and small off-white strokes strategically placed on a navy blue background. Roger's garb was not as complicated. He was handsomely dressed in a Cream jacket over a full black ensemble with his smooth textured shirt and silk tie.

My admirable view of my husband of two days was distorted by his demeaning stare and accusatory words that came across the table. "How did they know it is our honeymoon?" he said loudly, with his knife and fork pointing skyward as he rested his hands on the table.

I knew my attempt to be discreet in telling him to chill and just go with it would fail since everyone around us was now looking at the stars of the featured entertainment for the next two minutes or so. You know the look that your

The Cure Is In The Living

mother gives you when visitors are around, and you are not acting right, but she cannot admonish you with her voice; that is the only thing I could think of doing. In other words, I gave him the same stare he had given me earlier.

It was obvious that for the sake of appearances, Roger had mustered up a smile until the voice over the intercom continuing with his congratulatory announcement uttered, "so when you feel the ship rocking tonight, you will know who is to blame for it..." A wave of hearty laughter filled the room overtaking the previous clinging of eating utensils and glassware. I guess the church Elder was not appreciative of the implication of that statement because I got another weird look. I will give him that one, though, because I did not think it was that funny either, but the worst was yet to come; for Roger that is.

For a split second, as the group of colorfully dressed waiters and servers started in our direction in song and dance, I thought Roger was going to get up from the table. With a knitted brow coupled with a look of uncertainty, he shifted slightly away from the crowd, tossed his head back, and yelled, "Hell no!"

Now to my defense, I thought I had a valid reason to believe the worst here. If you calculated the months, yes months – not years, from our first meeting to now you would agree that I did not know much about this person so I was in the dark about how he would continue to handle this situation. But to my relief, he shifted back onto the chair, and once again, our eyes connected; and believe me, it was not a starry-eyed connection.

The feeling that had been stirring within me from when I witnessed Roger's first reaction toward our host's good jester on this special occasion, had now reached a point of explosion. As the performers came to the end of their act I could not hold my suppressed feeling any longer. With my head flung back extending the full length of my neck as if I was sitting in the dentist's chair about to have my teeth examined, I opened my mouth and expelled one of those 'I can't catch my breath' laugh. My hands were around my belly, and my knees moved further under the table with the edge of the crisp white tablecloth sweeping over my lap. Mustering some composure I pulled myself up and leaned forward as I wiped the tears from my eyes at the same time, trying to keep mascara from running down my face. Intermittently throughout the rest of the evening there would be an unexplained chuckle from me as I recall Roger's 'hell no' moment. Before long, he had no choice but to see the humor in it all and join in the laughter.

The Cure Is In The Living

Chapter 17

Laughter on Pause

At 6:00 a.m., I was at the cancer center almost three weeks after the wedding for that rescheduled follow-up appointment. What I liked about my team at the center was, while it might be a long day at times, they strive to keep your appointments on the same day. For me, it starts with blood work, then the scans, and a long wait before seeing the doctor who by then would have all your results. On this particular day, I was in my car heading for home by one in the afternoon.

There is this 'thing' that rises up within me when I should otherwise be afraid or troubled that causes me to be unyielding to the negative side of the matter. I was once again in that all familiar battle of negative versus positive emotions after hearing the results of that July 12, 2018 scan which read:

1. Interval increase in the size of a left lung base pleural-based nodule. Consider further evaluation with PET/CT.
2. Loculated fluid along the left aspect of the heart not clearly identified on prior exam.

In my language, it appears that the cancer had returned, but we needed more tests to be sure.

Obviously, the doctor was having difficulty determining what to say next since my expression was inconclusive. Eventually, he went with the generic, "It could be nothing, but I would like to proceed with the recommendation and do a full-body PET/CT scan."

My drive home that afternoon was horrible. I was so confident that I was doing well. It is nowhere near ten years since the last incident – how could it be back so soon. The next level of thoughts went to my future when it hit me.

"Oh my gosh - Roger!" I thought since it had not

been a month since my wedding. "Should I have tested before the wedding just to make sure I was still okay? No, I will be just fine. God would not bring happiness in my life now just to take it away within months." I said as I continued to convince myself that it could not be back so soon.

I was present for that PET/CT scan early on the morning of Friday, July 27, 2018. This time it was an in and out appointment. I would not see the doctor today because he did not have an opening, and they did not want to delay the test.

The results were to be available by the following Tuesday. When I did not hear from them, I adapted the 'no news is good news' attitude without concern even when a full week had passed since the scans. Plus, I was otherwise occupied with my busy workload at the office. But as another week was almost ending, uneasiness came over me, so I called the office, leaving a message that I have not received the test results. They asked to allow 48 hours for someone to get back to me, so I waited.

On the morning of August 8th, I telephoned Roger, who was already at work. I cannot remember what it was, but as I was ending the call with 'see you later' nonchalantly, he said, "Oh, by the way, my mother passed away last night."

"What?" I blurted. "Are you okay? why didn't you call me?" I asked.

"I figured I would tell you when I got home." He replied just as calmly as he spoke before. Talk about being cool in a time of trials; I had found my match.

By the weekend, I was back on the emotional battlefield, trying not to dwell on anything but a positive result. After all, there is no way they would wait two weeks if the cancer was back. Monday morning, I left another message and hoped they could hear the stern tones in my voice. Apparently, they did not because another 48 hours passed without a return call.

By now, arrangements were made for Roger to go to Trinidad for his mother's funeral. The morning of the 14th, before I took him to the airport, I called the doctor's office again. This time there was definitely a hint of frustration along with pleading in the message I left. I was on my way from work after 6:00 p.m., just a minute away from my house, when the doctor called. I knew something was wrong when the first question he asked was if I was in a position to talk. I took a deep breath and told him that I was. These PET/CT scan results read:

1. *Focal areas of metabolic activity within the pleural surfaces of the left hemithorax are increased in number and intensity since 2016.*
2. *New suspected metabolically active metastasis involving the right superior iliac crest.*

In my language, the cancer was definitely back on my lung, and a new spot was found on the right hip.

As I pulled into my garage, the question and answering session was still in play. The thought that the doctors had sat on this news for weeks came to mind several times, but there was no time for anger now. I just needed the facts surrounding my present condition.

Still seated in my car, I kept asking questions, desperately hoping that there was some good news he forgot to tell me. I needed answers based on facts because I did not want my mind free to formulate its own theories. I was about to go into my house to be alone with my thoughts, and I needed them to be moving in the right direction. Survival mode is that place where I always felt safe, and I had already flipped the switch to lift the barriers to protect my emotions. Still grabbing for a saving straw, I asked the question that halted the dialogue between the doctor and me. "So that is what, stage 2 or 3?" I asked.

"No, it is stage 4." He replied.

Seconds of silence followed. I was dumbfounded. First off, I have learned enough about cancer to know of the stages of the disease, the level of devastation, and the possible survival rates attached to each of them. Secondly, throughout my journey with lung cancer, I had always celebrated the fact that both times, the cancer was found at stages 0-1 telling me that there were great possibilities of survival.

To me, there would be a greater sense of hope if it was stage 2 or 3, but stage 4 – that was chemotherapy and pending death. I was so adamant about chemotherapy and stated in the past that it would be better for me to live like there is no tomorrow for the time I have left instead of being sick and in pain from medication. The awkward silence was due to the blow I felt deep in my stomach, causing a lump that seemed to be lodged in the base of my throat, rendering me speechless. In those few ticks marking time, it was as if my brain forgot to translate the message' swallow hard and breathe deep B.'

Feeling silly for asking a question for which I knew the answer, I apologized as he gave me his recommendations of a CT-guided biopsy of left chest wall abnormality and an MRI of my pelvis. I agreed for him to have the appropriate people call me to schedule the appointment. Then, I ended the call by wishing him a nice evening. As I gathered my things, exited the car, and closed the garage door, I knew survival mode would have to wait. I was not feeling anything –

Chapter 17—Laughter On Pause

good or bad, and I sure did not want to think anymore.

Roger called to check on me that evening, but I decided not to share the bad news. Burdening him while he was hundreds of miles away due to his mother's funeral would not be fair to him, nor would it bring me any comfort.

An appointment was set for August 30, 2018, for a biopsy of the lung area and an MRI to follow soon thereafter for the hip to determine if the spots were cancerous. Before the appointment, several doctors got together to review my case and decided it would be better to biopsy the hip area first, causing the cancellation of the lung biopsy. The new order was to perform a CT-guided biopsy of right iliac crest: Metastatic carcinoma (immunoperoxidase stains not yet performed, to conserve tumor tissue for molecular studies).

The doctor was expected at the hospital by 8 a.m., at which time I should be ready for surgery with all the necessary preparations completed. Fully clothed in my hospital garb and Roger seated across from my bed in the preoperative area, nurses and technicians came in with their own set of questions and as they fulfilled the procedures of their department. I had no objections to the questions – everyone was simply doing their job. The problem started when I was asked to voice my reason for being there that morning, and the nurse did not agree with me. "I am here to have a CT-guided biopsy of my right hip."

"We have here that the biopsy is for your lung." She said with confidence.

"No, that sounds like the old order. The new order for this morning is the biopsy of my hip," was my rebuttal with a 'here we go again attitude.'

As I looked across at Roger's face for support, I noticed disapproval instead and knew it was caused by my stern response. At this point, I did not care because it was I who has been in this position too many times. The dialogue continued since I knew exactly why I was there, and the nurse was certain of what was stated on her computerized order.

Eventually, with noticeable frustration, she politely told me that she would go back and check the orders again and get back to me. There was no doubt that she was reading the order she had correctly, so my suggestion was to call the doctor to find out what the order is since what is on the computer is different from what I am expecting. She responded that she would do that and left the room.

Within minutes two other ladies were walking towards my bed, but the Caucasian nurse that was attending to me from the time I got there was not among them. The leader was an African-American nurse who obviously was apprised of my resistance. It actually felt like security was called to remove me from the building for being a nuisance, except they were dressed in scrubs and surgical caps. She did not ask why I was so adamant; instead, she started to speak to me as if I was being a problem by not allowing the nurse to continue with the preparation necessary for a lung biopsy. Apparently, everyone had a schedule to keep, and I was holding up progress.

"Did you call the doctor to confirm the order?" I asked, ready to take her on as well, determined they were not going to manipulate me. Their answer was no.

"Is the preparation for the lung biopsy the same as the hip biopsy?" Again the answer was no.

"Well, then we will have to wait for the doctor because both he and my doctor told me the biopsy today is for my hip and not my lung."

Why am I being so stubborn? When the doctor who was going to do the procedure called to inform me of the

Chapter 17—Laughter On Pause

change in plans, I asked why and he gave me an explanation. So the way I understood it was that after he reviewed my scans and reports, he surmised that if the spot on the hip, a known place for lung cancer to metastasize, was cancerous, then there wouldn't be a reason to do another biopsy of the lung. That would mean the cancer had returned. He also said that was how he explained it to the Thoracic doctors to convince them to change the order of events. No one likes a non-compliant patient. For that reason, I was not surprised when everyone left my bedside, displeased with my attitude. And frankly, I still did not care. Knowing that I had discussed what needed to happen in length with the doctors before this appointment gave me the confidence to stand my ground.

Let's be clear; I was not rude to the nurses during this ordeal. Stern - yes, but rude – no. When this is all over, I did not want anyone to feel anger against me. After all, I will be passed out and at their mercy in a few minutes. Instead, this should awaken them to listen to the patient. Not everyone has the confidence or the fight left in them to stand up for themselves. If I did not ask the questions, if I was not sure of what I understood to be the process, I can easily be one of them. You and your loved ones are the greatest advocates for your well-being. Can you surmise why a patient who goes in for a surgical procedure is now being asked why and what they are there to get done? Yep, it's due to the number of sentinel events over the years. Some lost healthy body parts due to surgical errors. I can say I have witnessed some improved changes over the years. When I was having surgery on my left lung, they asked me which side the surgeon should be working on; then they had me touch the side, mark it, and had me identify again that they marked the correct side on which they would work.

It was a few minutes after 8 a.m. when a young man

with a dark complexion, straight shiny black hair, and a full beard entered my curtained cubicle. Yes, I noticed that this was our first meeting, and I know I would not remember his name.

"Good morning Mrs. Thomas," he said, as he continued to introduce himself as the doctor who spoke to me days earlier and the one who would be performing the biopsy. "I am aware that there was a mix-up with the order, and you are not crazy." He said, displaying a crooked smile.

I took a glance in Roger's direction, looking for an 'attagirl' expression but got nothing. With my full attention back to the doctor, I heard him say, "Someone did not update the system to show the change, but I am the doctor who ordered the procedure and am quite sure as to what needs to be done. Everything is now updated, and the nurses will be coming by soon to get you ready for the CT guided biopsy of your right hip".

"THANK YOU!" I exclaimed with an 'in your face' attitude. It was not the feeling of victory from the fact that I was correct but instead annoyance because it happened in the first place.

Four days later, I received the results that the biopsy proved to be cancerous, confirming that I had stage IV lung cancer metastasized to my right hip. The next step would be to meet with an oncologist to figure out the best type of treatment. Until that appointment, it would be me and the internet, trying to find information so that I would have the right questions or have some degree of understanding about my condition.

Roger and Mikey accompanied me to that appointment. My Oncologist, Dr. Saltos, was slightly balding but a very young doctor. Mikey voiced his concern that he looked

Chapter 17—Laughter On Pause

very young and might lack experience. He was also very soft-spoken in a nerdish way, which was a good thing to me; that meant high smarts and low arrogance. But the icing on the cake came when he said, "I would not recommend chemotherapy for you."

It no longer felt like a doctor-patient relationship; he became an instant friend. The barrier was down, and I was comfortable speaking with him without trying to convince him of what I think is best for me. On the back of my copy of the test results, he wrote three words in this order as possible treatment options.

1. Chemotherapy
2. Target Therapy
3. Clinical Trial

He explained that these would be the options for someone at my stage of lung cancer, but before they can make a definite decision as to which is best, he would like to do a cancer DNA. He also said that someone from the Clinical trial department would be available to speak with me that morning, so I said sure. That young lady made me more confused than I needed to be. At the end, I feared having to risk taking a placebo or a medication they are not sure of when I think I am dying.

When the doctor returned to close the meeting, I asked about my life expectancy for stage IV cancer patients, especially if they do not do any type of treatment. He gave me his disclaimer and made it clear that he does not like to focus on mortality rates, but without treatment, it could be within four months and with treatment nine months.

After the meeting, I was sent to the lab for a specific type of blood draw with results to follow in a few days. I set my next appointment to discuss those results and recommendations for September 21, 2018. I knew I would be back to being in attendance by myself. As serious as this had become, the unknown was too high for anyone to start missing work so early in the game.

I scheduled a second opinion with Mayo Clinic in Jacksonville, Florida, for October 15 and did the only foolproof thing I knew – take it to the Lord in prayer. I was overwhelmed, but my faith had never wavered. I believed my life still had a purpose, and this diagnosis was just a bump in the road. This, however, did not mean I give up doing my part in the fight for my life; I just could not do it without the one who created me and knew what would be best according to his purpose.

Statistics are what they are, but as I prayed, I could accept God's will for whatever time He had ordained for me, and I am choosing to live doing his command. If I was able to do that, I would win the battle. Still, I would need to fight to keep God at the forefront of my mind and not be pulled into a poor me mode.

One day at work, a member called me about a membership issue. He was a noticeable joyful gentleman, and we would communicate multiple times during the year regarding one matter or another. As I was responding to his inquiry, he made an unrelated statement that caught me off guard. In his Nigerian accent, he said, "I live my life to the fullest, Barbara. I work hard, and I enjoy my life." I mentioned how timely his statement was and told him I am trying to convince myself to do the same. Still not aware of my issue, he continued, "In my profession, I see patients of all ages who have died, and the reality is that there is a day that they were born and a day that they died. What is important when that

Chapter 17—Laughter On Pause

time comes is that IT IS WELL WITH OUR SOULS. Barbara, is it well with your soul?"

"Yes," I said, holding back joyful tears. It was then that I revealed my diagnosis.

"Okay – if it is well with your soul, just live your life."

Life starts looking different through life's binoculars. Just months before, I would not give a second thought in saying, *I will make a note and call you next year*, to my clients. Now, when similar situations come up, it is counteracted with 'don't make that promise, you might not be here next year.' My prayers included me finding the way to handle those thoughts when they arise. During one of those prayers, I heard that whisper in my spirit, 'Though he slay me, yet will I trust in him: but I will maintain mine own ways before him.' Job 13:15 (KJV). I was constantly reminded of a revelation through the word from Psalm 118:17 (KJV); "I shall not die, but live, and declare the works of the Lord."

Being a private person, the times that I have been battling cancer, only those very close to me were knowledgeable of intimate details, so imagine my surprise when that same spiritual whisper told me to tell the church about my condition. I did not want to and thought about not doing it. One of the reasons was a self-inflicted embarrassment. Because the diagnosis and my wedding were so close, I wondered how many were probably saying I knew before I got married but said nothing. The fact that I really did not know before the wedding did not make a difference; it was the thought of anyone talking wrong about me that mattered most. How sympathetic can we be when we allow a perception to rise above the truth in our hearts?

Before Sunday rolled around, God brought it to me again. This time there was a reason. He told me the congregation needed to know before I get evidence of my healing so that they will see that God is still real. I still was not there yet, though; now my new way out was they are going to say I was lying and did not hear from God.

I struggled with my pride for several days. Sunday morning – testimony time came, and I sat down fighting with my thoughts. I knew I was being disobedient and would regret it if I did not share what I was told. Reluctantly I took the microphone, and immediately my fears disappeared as I relayed the message. I could hear gasps across the sanctuary and saw a few hands covering their opened mouths in disbelief. In the end, I solicited everyone's prayers, not for healing but that no matter the time I have left on this earth, that time would be spent doing God's will – regardless of the outcome.

In my flesh, I was still trying to evaluate which treatment I should choose but found too many variables and unanswered questions. So I went to God, the one who knew it all, and asked to make it plain without a shadow of a doubt which treatment is the best one for me.

September 21st took forever to come but was worth the wait. Dr. Saltos reported that the test results showed what he suspected. I tested positive for 'EGFR exon 19 deletion mutation' and learned that a very small percentage of patients with non-small cell lung carcinoma have this mutation. His words brought great concern, especially since this was considered rare, but to my surprise, it was good news. The fact that I had the EGFR mutation meant that chemotherapy was not a good option, and it also disqualified me from the case study. There was only ONE option left on the table – Target Therapy.

The Lord had spoken – my prayers were answered, and I did not have to make a choice. Another amazing thing was the drug Osimertinib was approximately two (2) years

Chapter 17—Laughter On Pause

on the market and was a 1st line therapy. This meant I was allowed to use it even though I had not done chemotherapy in the past as required by other similar treatments. The side effects were minimal since the medication targets the bad protein and not the body as a whole. The other benefit was that all I needed to do was take one pill once per day.

I agreed for Dr. Saltos to order the medication, which had to be obtained through a specialty pharmacy. I swallowed my first tablet on Sunday, October 7, 2018, at 6:00 a.m. There would be a 60-day follow-up with blood work to see how the medication was working for me. Until then, I set my alarm to go off at 6:00 a.m. every morning to remind me to take one Tagresso table at the same time each day.

We all joined Nathan and his wife Ashley for Thanksgiving in Ocala that year. That Christmas season would be celebrated at Mickey's, and he intended to do it big that year. I knew in my heart of hearts it was because of the unknown elements regarding my health, and he wanted to make it 'my' big Christmas.

My train of thought was along the same lines as Mikey's. I felt like doing something special for my birthday. Not knowing what healthcare expenses might be ahead, I still could not simply throw caution to the wind – I had to be sensible. My 59th birthday was on December 10, and that special gift ended up being tickets for a trip to Virginia to visit my sister and her family. That plan caused the 60-day follow-up for December 7 to be rescheduled for November 30, 2018, a week earlier.

Fifty-four (54) days after starting my target therapy treatment, I was back at the cancer center being poked with needles for blood draws and IV, hooked to a heart machine, experiencing the weird feeling of contrast dye as it rushes through my body and the dreaded CT machine.

The Cure Is In The Living

Once again, I was sitting by myself in a waiting room full of other cancer patients waiting to hear how the cancer had behaved since the last time we were there. As I looked across the room, I did not see one person crying or appearing any more concerned than having a regular annual checkup. But the reality was that after that sit-down with the doctor, it would boil down to no change, decrease or increase; I wondered which one it would be for me today.

My hour and a half waiting room ordeal had ended as I was led to a room to wait a few more minutes for Dr. Saltos to appear with his usual greeting and formalities. He started with my blood work results, which came back with no changes from the previous results. My heart was fine as well. He shifted the papers and spoke very slowly. I kept a smile on my face to convince myself that I am not worried. 'Is he building up to something? Why not give me the scan result first? What difference would it make, the facts are on that paper in his hands, and nothing will change what's printed there – just blurt it out. I don't need the buildup.' I wondered as he continued to look through the pages.

Then finally, I heard the words, "The Tagresso seems to be working. The spots on your lung and hip are gone. The one on your hip had not only disappeared, but the damage cancer had caused to the bone so far is practically healed."

"Why didn't you tell me that first?" I said, amid an outburst of laughter followed by, "Thank you, Jesus!"

"Congratulations, I will see you again in three months," and my visit ended.

The only thing I could do was to keep whispering, 'thank you, Jesus.' I could not think of calling anyone until I got into my car. My first call was Roger, who I knew would be heading home by now.

Chapter 17—Laughter On Pause

"Hey, I am leaving the center now and on my way home," I stated calmly.

"Okay, what did the doctor say?" Roger asked.

When I got to the point that there was no evidence of cancer, I heard a scream like laughter I had never heard before from Roger followed with. "I told you, I told you God healed you. I knew it, I knew it."

We continued talking for a while, explaining the rest of the miracle, and ended with "okay, see in a few."

My subsequent calls were to my mother and then Pastor Neely, but I got their voicemails. New this good couldn't be left on a voicemail, so I figured I would try later. A few minutes later, the Pastor, who happened to be driving home as well, called me back. When I gave him the good news, you would have thought he won the lottery. He was shouting and laughing and praising God. "Yes, yes, yes!" he exclaimed.

Up to this point, I heard it, but it had not fully sunk in. Knowing I would be alone when I got the results, I had a layer of protection within me that would cause me to be strong, no matter the outcome. My faith automatically dictated that I give God thanks, but my emotional state was unchanged. My mission right now was to remain calm and make it home. But hearing the genuine joy and laughter from Roger and Pastor Neely, I started to feel the protective walls falling away slowly, and I truly began to feel blessed. Laughter is indeed contagious.

Again the words from Psalms 118:17 rang clearly in my thoughts 'I shall not die but live and will proclaim what the Lord has done.'

I waited until everyone got home before I contacted Mikey and Nathan because I knew they would have a ton of questions. My sons, who have been by my side since cancer interjected itself into our family, were in awe. Nathan could not comprehend my strength without acknowledging the presence of God in my life. His faith was being strengthened by the news. Mikey was overjoyed as well as he also could not contribute the good news to anything but God's presence in our lives. I spent several hours on the phone with them, going over what really happened and what the future looked like for their mother.

Sunday morning came quickly, and at the end of testimony time, I asked the church if they remembered when I told them that God wanted them to be a part of witnessing my miracle. Some nodded, others responded, "Yes," and some did not know what I was talking about. However, when I shared that my test results revealed no cancer in less than 60 days into treatment, the whole congregation cheered.

At the end of service, a woman confessed that her faith was wearing thin, and she honestly was wondering where God was during her struggles. With tears streaming down her face, she said, "Before you told us of your cancer returning months ago, I had asked the Lord to show me a sign that all of what I was doing is not in vain, and your testimony is the answer to my prayers. Thank you so much for sharing."

On the other hand, on 12/18/2018, another young lady straight up told me that she hated me. She shared that she could not even stand to remain inside the sanctuary when I was through giving my testimony, so she walked out. I remember seeing her when she left, but I would not have imagined she was mad at me. The 'why her and not me' question was so perplexing in her mind that she could not stand to look at me. By no means was I hurt by her confession. It presented an opportunity for me to share some of my experiences and how the Lord directed me through them and pointed out that He can guide her as well.

"My experiences did not always have good outcomes when measured by my standards, but because I believed Jesus is the author and finisher of my faith, I learned to accept the things that come my way," I assured her.

"So, how were you able to forgive?" She had asked after hearing a particular story. That was also another opportunity to speak about true forgiveness as I had learned it. The main thing is that forgiveness is not for the person who might have done you wrong; instead, it is for you to release the hate or anger so you can heal. Placing our problems at God's feet is the greatest thing we can do for ourselves.

When I was left alone to fight for my life after the first cancer diagnosis, I came to terms very quickly that I needed God to keep me alive more than I needed to be mad with anyone who had caused me pain. So it became my purpose to forgive.

Once again, I was reminded how life appeared unfair for me sometimes. Even when God rewards my faith in Him at the end of my trials, some might be offended because of the blessings extended to me. I wondered if they would endure or even comprehend the depth of the pain by God's grace I have endured before receiving those blessings.

The Cure Is In The Living

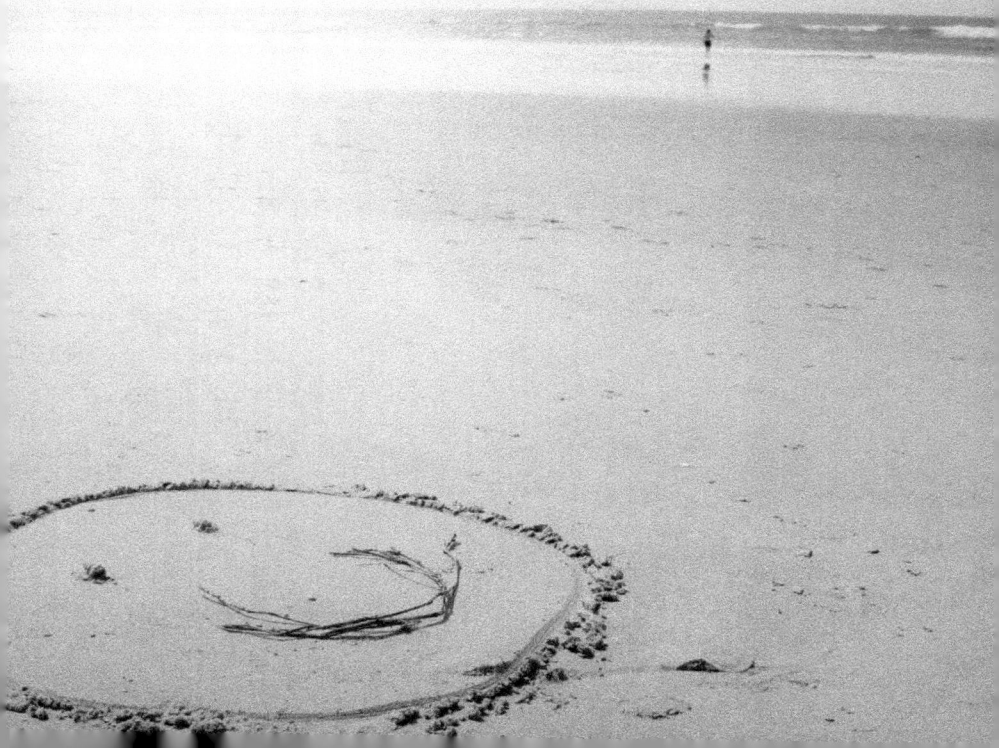

Chapter 18

BAMBA

When my Brother Dwight was diagnosed with cancer he was almost 44 years of age. By then I was seven years in - living with the stigma of a return episode. One might think that the disease made us immediate kindred spirits, but it did not. We did not view this as something that needed us to nurse it and be fearful of. We just had cancer and were doing what needed to be done to keep us alive and pity was not one of those things.

Dwight was a hard worker who ran his own trucking company for over 30 years. Treatment generated because of the illness was just something that slowed him down a bit but never brought him to a screeching halt. On the onset, he did chemotherapy and radiation followed by surgery to remove the tumor. After the initial surgery, they found out that the cancer had progressed more than anticipated which caused him to have a 2nd round of chemotherapy and radiation therapy. He told me one day that he was very creative in how he scheduled his appointments. He would make sure he did his blood work a few days before his doctor's appointment so that he would not have to sit around and wait for the results so they can determine his chemotherapy for that day. He had too much to do to be spending unnecessary time waiting for test results and doctors to make up their minds on what to do. He was very proud of his tactics.

We never voiced fear of the disease with each other. We just lived our lives. Our conversations were now discussions on politics, GMO, unhealthy meats, herbal teas to treat cancer, and the fact there does not seem to be anything safe to eat anymore. But we were going to do the best we could to stay healthy. He would send me posts now and then that addressed cancer healing properties or a doctor he heard about. I would check out everything he suggested. He did all the treatments recommended and after a while was cancer free. The routine then became a regularly scheduled blood test for his complete blood count (CBC) "Bawba, I am not doing this chemo again if the cancer comes back – it is hard." He told me shortly after completing treatment.

On one of his trips through Tampa, I happened to be in the hospital recovering from surgery. When he got there I already had another guest. It was then that I learned that my little brother was not shy but very vocal about his political opinions – I was very impressed. Not because of his in-depth knowledge but of his boldness and passion for the injustice he felt about our Government and upcoming election. He came to visit me, but he and my friend (a politician in her own right) were sharing thoughts for most of the visit. I was still in ICU and it was just a little more than 24 hours after lung surgery and I couldn't talk much – so that worked out well. His presence was good enough for me.

I view it as priceless because I would not start to discuss politics with anyone that I did not know their views first. I am a people pleaser – remember? While I would carry on a conversation with someone that shared my views, if they didn't, I would have nothing to say. Dwight had not met Gloria before he walked in that Intensive Care Unit – he knew nothing about her and that did not stop him one bit. I was silently proud of his boldness.

Until 2016, we had not kept in direct contact with each other much. We knew about each other's lives through our mother, but that one on one was not there and we decided to change that.

About 8 months after surgery we had a family gathering at Dwight's house and I spent the weekend. I still did not trust to drive myself for the three hour trip so we connected in Orlando and I rode with him in his 18 wheeler truck to his home in Okeechobee Florida.

Chapter 18—Bawba

That was a trip I will always cherish because it was the last such trip I had and the longest we had conversed in over 20 years. As you might guess, cancer was the main topic. We shared the things we learned about Genetically Modified products, the unsafe and unhealthy things he witnessed over the years he hauled produce and livestock from state to state. We talked about foods no longer in my diet and exchanged information we had on the herbal teas we had tried and those we heard about but not tried as yet. Yes – yes including Marijuana.

It was just a short time before medical Marijuana would become legal in Florida. In my research on cancer cures over the years though I had watched several documentaries about its healing properties and was already trying to figure out if I needed it along the way – how I could get the 'real' hemp oil.

Knowing Dwight would be shocked about me even thinking about it, I shared with him the information I found regarding the product's medicinal effects on pain and cancer. My brother being the matter of fact person that he is said, "Hey – I can get some for you if you want." He said laughing.

My response, "Nah, I wouldn't want either of us to get in trouble." The fact is I would have been a nervous wreck driving back to Tampa knowing I had marijuana in my possession. It would be all over my face that just passing a cop would make him suspicious of me and pull me over. I know that was silly – but nevertheless remember I do not like confrontation. I refused the offer.

We had a good chat that evening and at the end of it all we determined that there is nothing safe to eat anymore so what are we to do but live our lives the best way we can.

Florida Medical Marijuana Legalization Initiative,

also known as Amendment 2, was approved by voters in the Tuesday, November 8, 2016 general election in the State of Florida. Now the playful conversation was how to get medical cards.

We chatted now and then – the birthdays, holidays and occasionally – "hey – just checking on you" text and calls over the years that followed. As much as we tried not to go back to not keeping in touch anymore we did not succeed.

When I told him of the stage 4 lung cancer and me not wanting to take chemotherapy I thought somehow I would get his support on my decision. After all, he had told me in prior conversations how difficult it was – worse than the disease as a matter of fact, and that he would not do it again.

To my surprise he told me that I had to do what I needed to do – "cause trust me, even though I said I wouldn't do it again, when the time come, who knows."

Over the next couple of months, he would tell me that he was losing weight but his numbers are coming back okay. Before long he started a bad cough and that was also overlooked by the doctors as possible Bronchitis?

The results were that the cancer which he thought was at bay, had metastasized in multiple places. I was so angry that I forgot to feel sympathy for where he was. I was angry at the doctor's and our healthcare system. How can someone treating "cancer" patients complaining of certain symptoms like unexplained weight loss and persistent cough not get suspicious.

Now, I do not have a medical degree, but my ability in searching the internet tells me that rectal cancer that metastasizes, most commonly, would spread to the kidney and lungs. So it stands to reason, an already established type 3 cancer patient with unexplained weight loss and a massive cough should have warranted a scan despite the numbers from the blood test. Especially since the DNA of certain cancers presence is not always detectable through a blood test.

The first time Dwight told me of his unexplained weight loss and coughing, my immediate question was, "When is your next scan?" But he was not thinking of the possibility of the return of the cancer because his blood count was ok and he trusted the doctor.

One day jokingly I told him that worst case scenario, we both go to one of those out of the way cancer treatment centers; we can share a room and an IV stand but we are going to fight this.

Something happened during the beginning of 2019; we texted each other Happy New year wishes and then I missed a call on January 31ˢᵗ. That was the last text, because Dwight just stopped communicating with me and would not answer most calls and text.

I was in a different place than my brother. I wanted to know everything simply because over the years I have experienced that Doctors are not perfect. I questioned them for the things they might consider silly, I take it to be important – it was my life. So most naturally when I spoke to my brother I asked my brother questions as to what the doctor said. While that was comforting for me to know – it was intimidating to Dwight. He was a proud man and probably thought asking questions meant he would be viewed as inferior. I figured, having to answer questions from a nosy sister was something he could do without. I gave up on my periodic calls and texts after my Happy Father's Day wishes went unanswered. In my heart I felt at peace; I never thought his reason was intentional.

For some, praying for healing switched to concern

and hope that his soul was right with God. Yet in me somewhere, I kept thinking, God can turn this around and give
Dwight a testimony of his goodness and mercy. There must
be something else that can be done.

I did not speak to my brother until July 8, 2019 - It
was his birthday. The call was not generated to wish him a
happy birthday, but unknowingly, it was a step towards healing our relationship. It was not until I was several words in
before I it was Dwight on the other end. He told me that he
was strong and cancer was not going to get him – he was going to fight it. I wished him a happy birthday and exchanged
a few more words before ending the conversation. Even at
this juncture I was thinking the phone was enough, keep it
simple, don't overcrowd him. A physical visit was not in my
mind. I heard that he had lost so much weight that we could
pass in the halls and I would not recognize him. With that, I
decided I wanted to remember him as my brother and not as
a cancer victim.

He was in and out of the hospital several times after
that phone call. Mom was by his bed as she had been each
time he was hospitalized. On one occasion while mom was
speaking with someone with the same first name as mine, my
brother inquired if she was speaking with "big sister." A simple question to most but to me, it made me realize – he and I
were ok. I also surmised that while I was thinking that my
presence would not make a difference to him, I was wrong
even to the point of being selfish. I must be able to deal with
my memories which are minor to what my visit might mean
to my baby brother during this time of his life. I told my
mom I will be there to see him the following weekend.

On July 27, 2019, with my oldest son Mikey by my
side, we cautiously approached the room not certain what to

expect. The man was sitting in bed doing paperwork. I recognized him straight away but it could be because he was in the bed and not in the hallway. As I approached him, he stretched out his hand and held mine for a few seconds longer than a regular handshake. He then greeted his nephew as he put the paper and pen to the side. Without hesitation and questions from us, he immediately brought us up to speed on what had been going on. He pointed out that what looked as if he was sporting a Mohawk haircut was not deliberate at all. The clean shaved areas, perfectly symmetrical on both sides of his head, was a result of radiation treatment that he received to treat the latest tumor they found on the right side of his brain.

Trying to run down the list in his head, he paused and questioned himself, "What else? I think that is all of it. The worst part is knowing it's coming to an end but not knowing when." We were updated with months of suffering, pain, and uncertainty for tomorrow. One by one he spoke of the dates that doctors had predicted he had and those he had passed. He had that strong roughness about him still "Mi still deh ya, God is good." he chuckled; translation "I am still here, God is good."

"Amen to dat," was the only fitting response that I could think of at the moment.

The very next sentence was back to business. "Hey, I am looking for someone who auctions cars. I really want to get my son a car if it is the last thing I do," Dwight continued.

I immediately picked up my phone and texted my friend Gloria and got the contact information for an Auto Broker in Ft. Lauderdale.

"Thanks, I really want to get him a car," he replied.

By then, he had returned to his paperwork, answered

a few phone calls, apologizing for not having what they needed - but he was working on it. It was enough for my son to ask the question, "So uncle Dwight, you don't have anyone to help you with all this?" His eyes never left the paper as he raised one side of his lip, slightly followed by a mild chuckle, and replied, "No, it's just me," as he continued to draw lines across the paper, creating what looks like a scheduling grid.

His lunch came in, he looked up at the young lady and told her thanks, then went back to his papers. A few minutes passed when my son asked him if he was not going to eat before it became cold. He lifted the lid to see what was being served for lunch and commented it had no cheese and put the lid back in place. Mikey, being the 'get her done' person he is, jumped up and said, "I'll get you some cheese," and headed through the door.

The phone rang. He gave his apologies again. He mentioned that he was back in the hospital but working on it. The phone rang again and again. All the calls were business related. Each time, he would go back to his sheet of paper, drawing and filling in grids. Then out of nowhere, in a time of silence, with his eyes still on his paper, he said, "All people concerned about is what they need from me and not how I am feeling." It came from a place of such depth that I could not utter an answer. I just made a sound, "hmm."

Mikey came back into the room bringing a bowl of shredded cheese and obviously perplexed as he complained of the lack of service in the cafeteria. Apparently when he asked for the slice of cheese, they would not give it to him because the cafeteria was closed, and the register was too. So after trying to convince them of the importance of getting the cheese, he was turned down. Glimpsing the salad bar being

Chapter 18—Bawba

prepared, he went over, grabbed a coffee cup, scooped up some shredded cheese and said to the disagreeing young lady, "So I guess this is free." His uncle needed cheese for his hamburger, and by golly he was going to get it.

Dwight was growing noticeably tired as he rubbed his head in a circular motion, and gently laid back in the bed. He was waiting on his son who was on his way to visit and was anxious about him not being there as yet. "Bawba, call them for me and see where they are," Dwight instructed. "Sure," I replied.

I was able to reach the driver and reported that they were about 30 minutes away. "Thanks," he replied in appreciation. He closed his eyes - hands still on his head, papers on his lap, his briefcase at his feet, and the phone ringing.

It was now almost 2:00 p.m. and Mikey and I had not eaten. "Hey Dwight, mi soon cum back – wi a guh get sup'm fi eat."

"Aw right," he responded, as we headed up the hallway.

I was admiring the modest garden and seating area through the glass on one side of the hallway, and wondered if we could put Dwight in a wheelchair and take him outside if just for a minute. Looking for a possible exit to the small courtyard, I glimpsed a familiar figure ahead of me.

"Hey there!" I shouted.

"What?" my son exclaimed, assuming I was speaking to him.

"Your uncle, Justin, just went up that hallway," I replied, pointing to another hallway branching from the one we were on.

A handsome young man dressed in sweatpants, a hoodie jacket, and earphones securely in place, noticed me commanding attention. Grabbing my brother's arm, the

The Cure Is In The Living

young man pulled him back as he pointed in my direction.

I could not believe my eyes as I got closer. "What's going on..everybody changing on me." His usually well shaped low haircut was now grown out and full twisted dreads. Anyway that fright was further compounded when I was introduced to the handsome young man who by now I had suspected to be my 17 year old nephew which I had not seen in almost 16 years.

As we hugged in greeting I could see a curious look on his face as he said, "Hi!" For him this was the first time he was meeting this aunt and his cousin. For all of us, it was the very first time we uttered a word to each other. Again, 16 years of 'what could have been' had already passed never to be regained. A few more awkward words were exchanged and a warning that we might want to go off premises to find something to eat. "Go straight out through the front, hang a left, and then another left at the light. There are a few restaurants down main street." We thanked him and off we went for nourishment.

We returned to the room to find Dwight barely awake and his lunch tray just the way we left it – untouched. Mikey got a chance to speak with his cousin about school and his desired colleges and gave him some wisdom learned from his experience as a sought after athlete and colleges.

We hung around for another hour after Dwight had fallen asleep. I took a long look at him as we prepared to leave for home. I had no anxiety or regret of seeing him "that way." All I saw was my brother in a hospital bed and a hope that he will recover. He was still there three days later when my younger son went to visit and I was glad they both came to see him; since it was their last.

Chapter 18—Bawba

On the evening of August 15, 2019 the dreaded decision leading up to a transfer to Hospice was about to happen. The way I understood it, his pain had now reached a
level that the hospital could no longer effectively manage
and they had already given up hope of cure so... he was being transferred.

Mom has always had a mistrust of Hospice and un-
derstandably so. In her role as Pastor, she had accompanied a
few of her church members to hospice and had tried to defend the weak individuals who were not able to defend themselves. To her they were an institution of killers and so she
was adamant that Hospice is going to kill her son before the
Lord was ready to take him.

The reality that transportation was on its way to take
Dwight to hospice hit her like a brick. She knew it was going
to be too hard to watch and decided to say her goodbyes before they arrive. The anger, fear and finality all mixed into
one was evident as she leaned over her youngest son to bid
him farewell. Her weakened knees seemed to buckle slightly
under her seventy-four year old slender body as she laid
across her son's chest in tears. She had to get out of the hospital before Hospice came in.

I drove back down to visit him in Hospice the following Saturday. "This is Dwight's big sister Bawba ... the one
you have heard him talk about that she sort of raised him."

We did the handshakes, nice to meet you routine and
automatically turned my attention back to my brother..he was
asleep. I tried to focus on my brother laying there with subtle
groans. He appeared more rested than when I saw him last in
the hospital. He did not appear to be in much pain and was
sleeping quite peacefully. We did not talk much that evening
as guests came and went throughout the evening. When it
came time to be cleaned up for the evening, I left.

The Cure Is In The Living

Monday morning I arrived at my brother's bedside to find him in good spirits. "Hey, Bawba," he greeted me immediately.

"Hey, you looking good this morning" I responded, pleased with what I saw.

"He did good last night and this morning he even fed himself breakfast," Sonia shared.

I grabbed his frail outstretched hand and told him he was looking good but he ignored my words

"I am so glad you are here, big sister," and with deep emotion he repeated the sentiment.

"I am glad I am here, too," this time looking away. He said it again, "I am so glad you came." All the time holding onto my hand. I scouted the room looking for a chair so that I could sit and continue holding his hands but did not see one.

"Hold a sec, I will be right back" I told him as I left the room to find a chair.

As I placed the chair by his bed, held on to his hand closest to me, he reached over with his other hand and rubbed the top of my head. "I love you Bawba, I am glad you are here." And there I sat for the next couple of hours talking, singing and reading the Word for him.

As visitors came in and out, Dwight was able to address everyone by name. He was noticeably tired but would not go to sleep. He would doze off for a few, then hear a sound and would be wide awake.

As I was feeding him lunch I chucked about me feeding him and he smiled as well "you fed me when I was a baby and you feeding me again now"

"Look at that, you are right" I said in agreement.

After a while, his wife had left to run a few errands

and I settled in a nearby recliner to do some work on my computer. Ever so often, I would resume my place in the chair closest to his bed when he seemed to be in discomfort. He would occasionally ask me how I was doing, and if I am ok. He questioned me about my phone, if it is still working; he had given me that phone several years prior. At one point he said to me, "what am I doing in this place, I am getting out of here and going home soon."

"Ok then, I will believe that with you." And I truly had hope that his fighting spirit would prevail.

On August 20, 2019, while he was still at the Hospice facility, Dwight's closest friend Tony and his Pastor came by for a visit. As I was being introduced, Tony stated, "Yes, I saw you at the hospital." For a brief moment, I smiled but thought he was mistaken because I did not meet any of Dwight's friends while he was in the hospital. "Me?" I responded. "Yes, you had on a purple dress. We passed each other in the hallway – you looked at me with this odd look..." I still hesitated because I do not own a purple dress.

Then I remembered, "Oh, yes. Hello." It was the tall slender man I passed in the hospital hallway the week before. For clarification, the dress was blue.

Dwight was in a deep sleep and we were not able to wake him up all morning. Tony tried several times... "Hey buddy, wake up man." But Dwight was so drugged that he would not respond.

Eventually Pastor Ruskin pointed out that when the thief was on the cross and asked Christ to remember him when Christ came into his Kingdom, Christ did not ask him any questions about his past or told him to do anything. All Jesus said was, "Today you shall be with me in paradise." So we don't have to wake him up to talk. Pastor Ruskin divulged that he had a very good spirit filled, salvation oriented conversation with Dwight a month or so ago. From that conversation, he sincerely felt that Dwight was in a good place spiritually.

Pastor Ruskin stood looking intensively at Dwight for a bit as if it was only the two of them in the room before he started praying. As Pastor Ruskin paused in praying for Dwight, he told us that he did not believe that this was the final place for Dwight; that He believed that Dwight was going to get well and would have a great testimony regarding his healing. His words validated my outlook on the situation as well and thought God was really going to move – against the odds. Pastor Ruskin had a stipulation however and that is – we must wholeheartedly believe Dwight would be healed and that extended to everyone who cared for him or visited him. I took comfort in his words as it added a little more to my hope as well.

Dwight's guests were surprised to learn that I had been inflicted with cancer as well, yet I appear not to be bothered by it. I assured them, I was not affected by my brother's state although I know this could be me someday. He offered to pray for me and I happily accepted. Now it is a known fact that we should not allow every and anyone to pray for you, I felt a peaceful spirit with the three visitors.

I left for home late that afternoon, knowing my sister would be there the following morning. By the time I made it through traffic and got home, I was so tired. All I did was shower and hopped into bed. As I laid there, curiosity got a hold of me, and I grabbed my phone to see where exactly and how far Tony's church was.

I was back at Hospice shortly after 1:00 a.m. Saturday morning August 24, 2019, after receiving a call at 10:00

Chapter 18—Bawba

p.m. Friday telling me he might not make it till morning. Standing by the side of his bed – his eyes looked distant, but little by little as I talked to him, it was apparent that he was looking directly at me. As he struggled to speak, I tried to convince him that he did not have to say anything. But he kept trying to the point I could see his tongue trembling as he tried to get words out. Just like a push of air and voice combined, he said, "whappen" – translation "What's up?" Those were the last words he spoke.

Regardless of what we wanted, hoped, or thought would happen, Dwight totally stopped breathing some time after 4:50 a.m in the wee hours of the morning of Saturday, August 24, 2019. It might have been seconds or minutes after mom, and I left the room to stretch our legs. It was almost as if he was waiting for us to leave the room; we were the only two that were still watching his every move. The same voice that announced in my ear "its cancer" over 12 years ago was the same voice that announced that morning, "Barbara, he is gone."

"No!" I shouted as a flood of different emotions came over me. Why did I leave the room when I did? I was not there with him. I did not see him transition. Yet none of that was more devastating than the fact that my hope, my faith that he would be better, had died with him, and that was final. I held back my emotions as I watched the others tearfully gathered around him. Now and then, I would hear, "Dwight is gone. I can't believe it; he is dead." As if my crying would have made a difference to my dearly departed brother, I exited the room into the hallway, leaned up against the wall, and started to cry. I could not hope anymore. I could not exercise faith anymore. The thoughts just kept coming. I could not recall at any other time in my life where something felt so final to me. My belief that prayer can change things was not providing any comfort in my grief. My baby brother was gone, and my hope was not too far behind if I am not careful.

Does that mean I was wrong in believing Dwight would rise up from his bed of affliction? I think what I felt was Dwight's strong will to live and I was now reminded that what we want does not always match God's purpose and will. While the cancer destroyed his body he never stopped living until God said so.

But now it's time to rest; sleep on my brother, God knows best.

Chapter 19

The Unexpected Detour

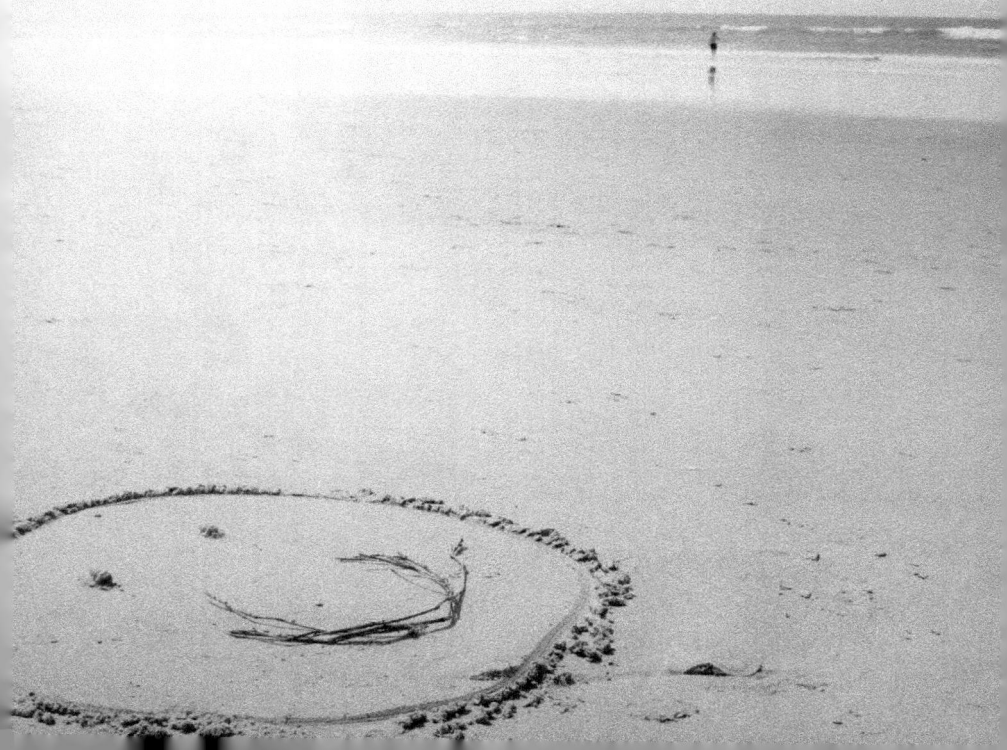

The beginning of 2019 started full of blessings. I was alive to witness the birth of Nathan's daughter – my first grandchild and also share in the joy of Mikey's wedding to Jen, his girlfriend of five years. To many people, such events can become second nature. To me, they were monumental; because I was able to rejoice and say, "God kept me!"

On October 31, 2019, I was on vacation in Georgia, and I felt a small scabbing on my breast. I also noticed it was a bit sensitive to touch. By November 6th, I was in the office of my Primary Health Physician. As he conducted his examination of my right breast, he did not need much information from me before he turned to his assistant and said, "It could be the very early stage of Paget's Disease."

Everything was okay until he said, "It's a type of breast cancer." There I was again, by myself, trying to be strong as I face yet another cancer appearance. Spoken words are as light as the breath used to give them life, but when it's bad news, those words surely weigh heavy on one's soul. Be strong, B; you will be just fine. I repeated quietly.

Dr. Michael Cromer is one of the best doctors I came across along my health care journey. He was so concerned about my peace of mind that he decided not to toss me to someone else and have me wait for days for another appointment. Instead, he chose to perform a shave biopsy himself right there in the office.

On the drive home, in an effort not to lose my composure, the self-encouragement continued, "Here we go again B – here we go again. We can do this." Talking to myself instead of God at this pivotal moment was not a lack of faith in Him; instead, it was 'me' that I did not trust.

Upon entering my home that afternoon, the pathway led straight to my computer. I needed to find out what in the world is Paget's disease because I needed to know what to pray for. This was the first explanation I found:

"Paget's disease of the nipple is a rare form of breast cancer in which cancer cells collect in or around the **nipple**. Cancer usually affects the ducts of the **nipple** first (small milk-carrying tubes), then spreads to the **nipple** surface and the areola (the dark circle of skin around the **nipple**)." June 22, 2019, breastcancer.org

As if that was not scary enough, I kept reading other articles. Some stated that about 80% of the time, there is cancer someplace else in the breast as well. Another said Paget's was very rare and represented less than 5% of breast cancer cases. "Things are not looking very good B." was my thought, but I knew nothing was final. Like times past, my internet searches always equip me with possible questions to ask my doctors when we meet in person. I had learned never to allow them to cause any anxiety.

On November 12, 2019, at 1:06 p.m., my life took another turn. The fact that the person's voice that I heard when I answered the phone was Dr. Cromer instead of a receptionist let me know that it would not be good news. "Your results came back, and it is cancer," he divulged as if he was confirming something I already knew. Gone are the days when doctors would appear hesitant in giving such news. We now have the 'rip the band-aid off' technique, which quite frankly is good for me. He also told me that this cancer had no connection to lung cancer. I now had two different cancers posing a territory war in my body.

After acknowledging that I heard him, he continued to make a few more comments and asked a question or two as if to figure out if my calm responses were genuine. He offered to have his office call me with recommendations for a few specialists if I did not already have one, and I accepted.

I decided to keep a previously scheduled November

Chapter 19—The Unexpected Detour

15th mammogram appointment at another institution. Deep down, I was hoping they would show whether or not there was another source of cancer from Paget's disease, as the article had suggested. My other reason was that the results would be available when I had my meeting with the Breast Cancer specialist, and I wanted to make sure I had as much information as possible beforehand.

The first official question the technician asked before starting the mammogram was, "Do you currently have breast cancer?" I told her about the Paget's disease diagnosis. She left the room to consult with someone and came back satisfied it was okay to proceed with the 3D mammogram. The 3D option apparently would have provided a clearer picture with more images being taken and from different angles. The mammogram increases doctors' chance of catching breast cancer early, especially for a patient with dense breast tissue. That was how the receptionist explained it to me, followed with, "I must tell you though that it cost more, and the insurance might not pay for it."

After the normal waiting period, the mammogram results came back normal, with no evidence of cancer. For some reason, though, the result did not give me a 'thank you, Jesus!' outburst as I would have liked it to. Instead, I had a 'something did not feel right' feeling. While I could accept that they did not find a cancerous cell to confirm the nature of Paget's disease of the breast, not acknowledging the presence of the Paget's gave me concern.

All the years of taking this test to detect the presence of breast cancer, I never thought it could be misleading. Now I know thinking that a mammogram is guaranteed to detect all types of breast cancer is a myth. The fact is, highly sophisticated technology or not, they all have their limitations, and mammograms are no exception – plus, human beings read the results. Come on now; no one is perfect; only God occupies that spot, so I am not upset.

My first meeting with the surgeon on December 5, 2019, was an interesting one. Dr. John Kiluk did not quite know what to do with me. It was not due to his intellect or knowledge of his profession, but our joint concern for my quality of life. My case was an unusual one. Dr. Kiluk's previous consultation with other doctors including Dr. Saltos, did not immediately provide a clear passage as to how best to handle my case.

One problem that does not usually present itself to most doctors is that I had two (2) unrelated cancers, of which one was successfully being controlled with medication. That means, to treat the breast cancer, they needed to find a way not to interrupt the lung cancer protocol. However, there seemed to be no way around putting a hold on the lung medicine that is working in order to treat the breast cancer. Even if I went with only surgery, I would have to stop taking the medication weeks before and after surgery to eliminate possible life-threatening problems. However, before we crossed that bridge, I had to face the first test scheduled for December 26, 2019, which was to have an MRI on both breasts.

Christmas that year was a simple yet busy one. I was to be the host, but my son Nathan was unable to join us in Tampa. So I prepared as much as I could on Christmas Eve with plans of starting at 8:00 a.m. for Ocala on Christmas morning to visit his family. It was his daughter Mya's first Christmas, and I was determined to spend some time with my granddaughter for her first Christmas.

Of course, Mya being my first granddaughter, meant there were gifts to be delivered as well, and I wanted to see her expression as she unwrapped them. After all, I was

Chapter 19—The Unexpected Detour

blessed to be alive to share that precious moment, and I was not going to toss it aside.

I was able to see her crawl and move around as she displayed her own opinions on what she did or did not want. Her cute response to the soft cuddly toy and intrigued with the flashing lights on the replica of a telephone was priceless. She did not show any interest in the outfits; she gave that privilege to her mom.

When the MRI results came back a week later, there was not only evidence of Paget's disease in the right breast – surprise! Just as the article had suggested, there was indeed another mass in the same breast. As if that was not enough for a woman to swallow, they also found a mass in my left breast. This determined the next test, which was an ultrasound-guided core needle biopsy of both breasts. That result ended up being fatty tissue in the left but definitely two locations of cancer in the right breast.

After the biopsy results and a meeting with the Tumor Board, my medical team's recommendation was mastectomy without reconstruction. In my language, the removal of my entire right breast. Surgery was scheduled for February 10, 2020. How did it get from simply removing only the area of Paget's disease to the removal of my entire breast? I could feel my strength leaking away.

This meant another visit to the internet – I needed a second opinion, and I needed it from the highest-rated cancer center in the nation that I could get to. I found that for 2019-2020, MD Anderson was ranked #1, and boy did I sing hallelujah when I found out that they had a center within their network just miles away in Jacksonville, Florida, Baptist MD Anderson. That trip I could afford; look at God.

The day before my 2nd opinion at Baptist, I received

a call from the breast specialist from Moffitt. They asked if I wanted to meet with the doctor before surgery since every conversation, except the first, had been by phone. I thought that was extremely nice of Dr. Kiluk and scheduled an appointment for January 24, which would be perfect since by then, I would have my 2nd opinion and would be able to either go through with the original plan or discuss another option.

I was hopeful as I arrived for my appointment to Baptist MD Anderson on Wednesday, January 22, 2020, for my second opinion. My team was a physician and her two assistants – all female. She recommended removing only the affected areas and reforming the breast with what is left. She was also pushing for me to have chemotherapy and radiation to kill any remnant of cancer that might be lurking in the area. She also stated that if I do not do the treatments, the lumpectomy might be a waste of time. On the topic of reconstruction, she said if there was enough fatty tissue in my tummy area, at a later date, the belly flap procedure could be used to reconstruct the breast. That sounded a whole lot better than using silicone implants.

"Not jumping the gun here, but I have more than enough flap on my abdomen for that procedure, and to get a tummy tuck in the process... where do I sign," I said jokingly, finally finding a crack in the solemn conversation for a bit of laughter. I need laughter when anxiety is trying to take hold.

Regardless of the recommendation of a less-invasive surgery, the other concerns were still the same. They would need to stop the Tagresso medication for about three months while they administer a chemotherapy and radiation protocol. "It was just your luck that you have two different cancers,"

Chapter 19—The Unexpected Detour

she said. My previous doctor had also referenced my situation as bad luck, and it felt as negative then as it did now. But this time, I was offended and could literally feel the words bouncing off me. I do not deal with luck; I deal with a living God who does not operate according to a human's views. If I don't make it, that has nothing to do with luck; I believe in God's will for my life, and I will not die before my time. I got the second opinion that I came for, so I thanked them and started my journey back home to ponder my choices. I was too overwhelmed at this point to make a decision right then.

As if I did not have enough, on Thursday, January 23, the day following my visit to Jacksonville, there was something else brewing that would test my strength. I was experiencing abdominal cramps a few hours after having some seafood soup for lunch. By 6:00 pm, it had increased in intensity that I was in bed with a hot water bottle on my tummy and sipping ginger tea. This had brought me relief over the past few months whenever I had experienced such cramping, but I was not getting any relief this time. The pain did not only get worse, but I was also severely nauseous, but nothing would come out. Could it be food poisoning, I wondered? I sat on the side of the bathtub with my face over the toilet, crying and asking God to let me throw up, thinking I would feel better, but nothing happened.

I went back to bed, but it became uncomfortable, so I tried the floor, which proved to be no better, so back to sitting on the edge of the bathtub. The self-diagnosing continued as I tried to find a cure to relieve the increasingly intense pain but to no avail. 'Maybe I should go to the emergency room,' I thought. I checked the time and dismissed the idea as I convinced myself that sitting in a waiting room in my condition would be worse than doing it at home.

The Cure Is In The Living

It was already after 9:00 pm when from that soft whisper within me, I heard the words' intestinal rupture.' It was so profound that it could not be ignored. What if I am being warned – could that happen? With my basic knowledge, I know that a perforated intestine can cause infection leading to sepsis. So the emergency room it is.

I had assured Roger, who was keeping me company earlier, that I would get over this and encouraged him to go to bed since he leaves for work at 5:00 am. Now as much as I hated to wake him, it could not wait. We both got dressed, and as we left the house, I knew my rule had to be broken when Roger asked, "what is the address of the hospital."

The reason for the inquiry was because I had told him numerous times not to take me to a hospital in the area where we lived because of other patient's experiences there. But that night, I was feeling so bad, and with the idea of sepsis swirling around in my head, we ended up at the same hospital. To my surprise, I walked into the emergency room and was seen immediately. I was still trying to answer questions in between hacking and groaning when Roger came in from parking the car. It was perfect timing because now they needed contact information, and I was not in a state of providing them. I sat in my wheelchair, waiting until all of Roger's questions were answered and for me to be assigned a bed.

A team of attendees came in to take my vitals and go over the reason for my visit. Between gags, I gave my account of events since noon that day. As soon as I was able to sit still long enough for them to give me a physical check, they gave me medication for nausea and took me off for a CT scan of my abdomen. "Oh no, not another scan!" I said out loud, but no one paid any attention to my babbling.

Chapter 19—The Unexpected Detour

I have often been told that I have inquisitive ears, and pain or drugs did not dilute that ability at all. I was barely back from radiology when I could hear a strained conversation going down the hall with someone trying to find the patient, Mrs. Morris. Somehow I figured that was me since the system had my other name on record. Since I had given them the new name when I came in a few minutes ago, I surmised everyone's electronic device had not been updated yet. It proved to be my doctor of the hour who was confused as to why the name she had in her notes did not match the room number. Before long, she was at the nurses' station asking for an update on Mrs. Morris in bay 400. The nurse was not helping the matter because he kept insisting that he did not have a Morris in that room and had no idea who or where she was.

"Roger, can you go and tell that lady right there that I am the person she is looking for," I said, pointing to the confused woman standing by the nurses' station.

As they both entered the room, I could see the questionable look on her face. "Mrs. Morris?" she said as she gestured for a handshake and introduced herself as the attending doctor.

"It's Thomas; we gave all the changes at check-in," I answered.

In all fairness to the doctors at this hospital, my hesitation regarding this hospital was never about the doctors, but the administrative inefficiency and long wait times. I am proof that good doctors can lose patients because of the staff at the front desk. Anyway, here I am – no turning back now.

The doctor attempted her apology again before revealing that the scan showed a blockage in my small intestine. After explaining what that meant and that I will be admitted, she further inquired as to which pain medication would work best for me. The only one I could recall without hesitancy was morphine, so that was the one I agree on having.

"Will I need surgery to remove the blockage?" I asked.

Her response to my question was vague, but I was comforted with her saying not necessarily since I already have the breast surgery coming up. "Okay, the nurse will be in to give you the morphine for pain and get you upstairs as soon as a room is assigned; hope you feel better soon." She said as she turned to leave.

I figured it was getting late, and there was no reason for Roger to stay, so I suggested that he go home and get some sleep. There was nothing more to be done for me, and he needed to be at work in a few hours. I remained in my screened room for a while until the nurse returned and added the pain medication to my IV as a young man appeared to take me to my room. Within seconds, It was hello morphine, good night all!

Roger called in to work late the next morning so that he could stop by the hospital first. The visit had to be short but appreciated.

The Hospitalist was my next visitor who confirmed the prior night's diagnosis, except she informed me that a surgeon would be in to see me that morning as well.

"A surgeon? I thought you could take care of the blockage non-surgically." I said frantically. All I could think of is I would have to stop the lung cancer treatment, and I have another surgery already scheduled in 17 days. I cannot have another surgery now. I did not have time to think because the doctor kept talking, trying to convince me the surgeon was just for observation. I felt like I was being played – with her fast-talking smiling self and extra comments about

Chapter 19—The Unexpected Detour

her time off the day before. She knew I had to have the surgery, but I was too drugged to call her on it.

Before 10:00 am, the surgeon was present with his assistant by his side. At first, he had not said anything I had not heard before. There were still two options to try first, but a decision was not yet made as to which one, and no one seemed interested in either. However, the surgeon's spin on the situation was that he would like to look at it with a camera if I would allow him to do so. In my drugged state, I did not know if I formulated in my mind that it would be like the endoscopies I had in the past where no cutting was involved or if he deliberately led me to that place.

Within an hour, a man came by to take me to surgery. This was moving way faster than I anticipated, and I had a mixture of thoughts swirling in my mind. 'Inserting a camera is not surgery – right' I questioned myself as I moved from bed to gurney. 'wait a minute, no family member knows I am going to surgery, and that cannot be good – can it?

The trip from a private room to a testing area has been one that I have taken many times over the years, and it still makes me feel awkward. I am always conscious of the people we roll by in the hallway, and I never know how to act. Do I smile or say hello? Or, do I pretend I don't see them in hopes they don't notice my messed up hair and hospital garb lying helpless in the hands of some youngster pushing my bed to someplace only he knows? After a few turns and even more double doors, I occupied a corner of the pre-op holding area.

My assigned staff was by my side in seconds, asking for my name and why I was there. That was a tricky question because I really was not sure, so I explained my situation, hoping they could come up with the right one-word explanation for the procedure.

"I am concerned that no one knows I am about to have surgery," I said to a beautiful young nurse with a noticeable Caribbean accent.

"Do you want to call someone – I can lend you my cell phone."

"My husband, but I cannot remember his phone number," I said, sounding as if I was drunk. Truth be told, it's not that I could not remember the number because I never took the time to know it. Yes, I am one of those who rely on my contacts listing on my phone.

"Okay, I will get his number from the system and give him a call." She caringly offered.

She completed her tasks of getting me registered in her area and walked off to fulfill her promise of contacting Roger. She had returned by the time they had a newly placed IV and blood drawn. She paused, just enough to dial the phone number she had written down, then handed me her cell phone. To my disappointment, I got the generic voicemail and left a message. Realizing my despair, she took the phone and pulled out her piece of paper again.

"Let me make sure I dialed the right number – 3528.."

I interrupted her before she could finish, "that is my phone number."

"But that is the number they have for your husband – let me double-check." And she was off again.

Sure enough, she was correct. The number they had for both of us was mine, and I knew for a fact, Roger gave them his contact information when we checked in. I remembered because when they asked for the contact person's name and phone number, I turned to Roger, who stepped up to the desk and provided the information. We now have two

Chapter 19—The Unexpected Detour

strikes; last night, they did not have the right name, now they do not have the contact information. Some of the reasons I was told not to go to this hospital was becoming real for me. In my case, these incidents were minor but could have more significant consequences if things were different. Thank God I was coherent enough to make my own decisions, and they did not need Roger to give permission for my treatment.

I dozed off again when I was awakened by a nurse who introduced herself as the nurse who will be with me during my surgery. I had to repeat for her who I was and why I was there. Slightly perturbed, she said thank you, looked towards the hallway, and asked, "Where is Frank with my..." I could not make out what Frank supposedly had that she needed to complete her task with me as I dozed off again. I cannot say that I enjoyed the effects of the morphine, but I was surely allowing it to do its thing.

By then, my Caribbean nurse was back, offering to find my husband's work number from the internet so that she can call him for me. I gave her the company name, and off she went on her mission to help me feel secure. The surgical nurse was still bothered that Frank was still not present, but I was half asleep, half awake, and came alert only when I heard my name.

"Okay, Mrs. Thomas, I am going to go ahead and start, and when Frank gets here, I can do that part." The surgery nurse said as she moved closer to the top of the bed.

Again she asked me to repeat my name, and I did. The next question was for me to confirm the procedure I was getting done. As I explained the procedure, she adjusted the white identification band on my wrist to see the name. She acknowledged my name matched the wrist band but tried to correct me when I told her the type of surgery I was there to get.

The Cure Is In The Living

The funny thing is, while I could not remember the medical terminology for my procedure, I knew without a doubt that what she said I was there to do was not it. The medical term begins with an E, and her word started with an S – it was that simple.

"I do not remember the correct name of the procedure, but I don't think it's what you just said." Once again, I explained that I had a blockage in my small intestine, and the doctor wanted to take a closer look with a camera.

She then pulled a paper out of her pocket and asked the question, "What's your name again?"

This time I forced myself to be as alert as I could be as I raised my head from the pillow and repeated my full name, just to hear her say, "So where is Mrs..." The name she voiced was neither my former or current name. 'I would muster a guess that she is with Frank, who you have been waiting on for the last several minutes,' I thought as she hurried away, noticeably embarrassed in finding out that she was with the wrong patient. Even with the seeming incompetence around me, I fell asleep again – the morphine was doing its job.

Next, I was awakened by a young man trying more than normal to assure me that he was my surgical nurse. He shared with me that he knew what happened earlier but not to worry because he was the correct assigned surgical nurse. The tone of his voice and the way he was trying to convince me that everything is now okay gave me the feeling that the young lady's action had caused a stir.

Everyone had done what they needed to do, and it was time to go to the big room. Again, I was experiencing the familiar sight of scrub-clad men and women with surgical head coverings and masks hanging around their necks. In this neck of the woods, those you pass in the hallway on your

Chapter 19—The Unexpected Detour

way to the cutting room do smile at you. I started to focus on the lights in the ceiling as, one by one, they disappeared behind me. "Here we go again, B, it is you and God."

My thoughts were interrupted by my Caribbean nurse's call, asking to speak to Roger Thomas as she swiped her card in the reader on the wall. As the door swung open, revealing the operating room, she repeated his name. In seconds, my gurney was lined up with the operating table, and in mid transfer, literally one leg on the operating table and the other still on the gurney, my Caribbean nurse handed me the phone. I could barely finish saying, "I am about to have surgery right now." When she took the phone and continued the conversation with Roger, the last thing I heard her say was, "give me your phone number, and someone will call you when the surgery is over." I was okay, now that someone else knew what was happening.

Everyone in the room identified themselves and their purpose there. IVs were checked, sheets and trays adjusted, and with a syringe in hand, my nurse announced that they were about to put me to sleep and that I should start counting 100, 99, 98, 97; I had to really concentrate, though – I didn't want them to think I cannot count backward.

I was awakened by someone calling my name, followed by "the surgery went well, and the doctor will be here shortly to speak with you." She barely completed her sentence when the surgeon walked in behind her with a broad smile as if he was very proud of himself; and he was. Taking a quick look around, I realized I was already back in my room.

"I am glad I went with my gut." No pun intended, I am sure, "You had a hernia where part of the small intestine broke through a weakened section of your abdominal wall and got stuck. It had caused a strangulation effect on a section of the intestines. He stressed that it was bad enough that he thought at first it was too damaged to repair. He was also in awe of how twisted my entire small intestines were, which he believed was caused by scar tissues from a previous surgery.

"But I was able to fix it and a few other things (which I never asked what those 'things' were). You should be okay now, and I will come by to see you tomorrow." Regardless, while the doctor felt that his gut-directed him to go in and fix my gut, I know it was my Lord who directed him.

This experience taught me something else about my body. Before the doctor left, he asked if I was feeling hungry, and it was then that I remembered that I had not eaten or drunk even water since the day prior, but I did not feel a bit hungry. When I told him no, he replied that it was okay and that my intestine would let me know when it is ready to process food. When that happens, I will feel hungry and can start with clear liquids. God's creation is so perfect.

I went back to sleep, and when I awoke, around 2:30 pm. I got my phone to make a few calls and saw a missed call from a New Port Richey 727 area code. As I listened to the message left, all I could do was smile. Someone from the hospital had left a message for Roger on my phone telling him the surgery was over, and I was in recovery. They still did not have my husband's number on file.

Feeling a hint of frustration creeping in, I took a deep breath and leaned back onto the bed with my eyes closed. To think, I could have died last night if I had not come to the hospital when I did. 'B, you are still alive. Thank you, Lord, for your saving grace."

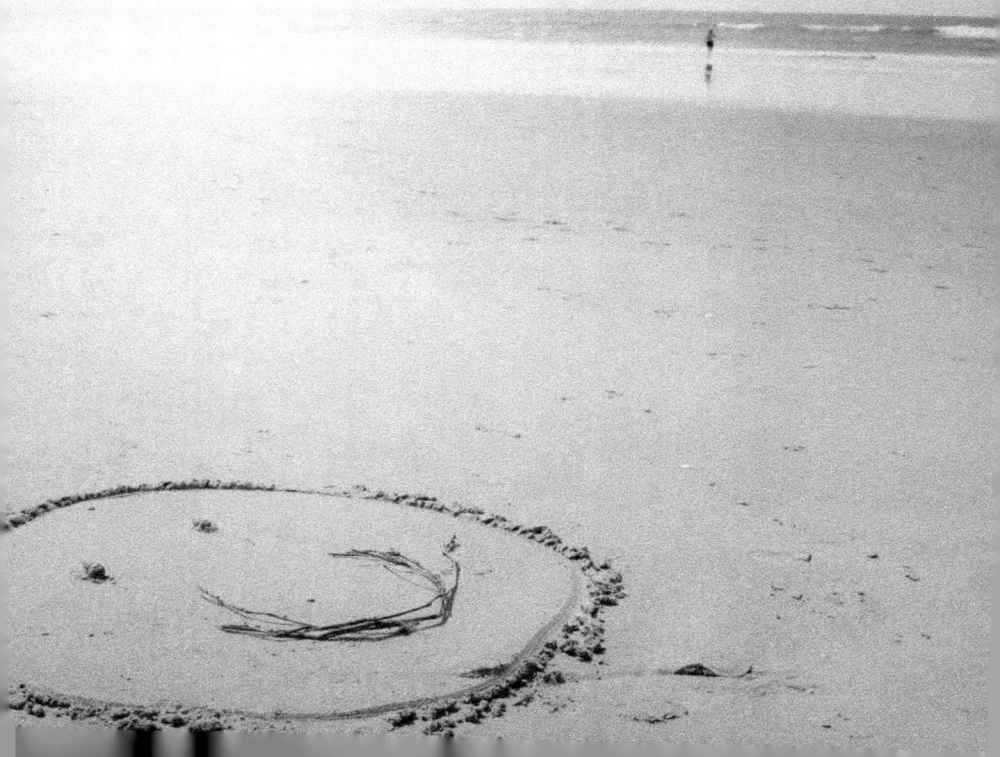

Chapter 20

Back On Track

Obviously, I could not sit down with the breast surgeon that afternoon at Moffitt, so we rescheduled for January 31, 2020.

"Oh, you poor thing," was the nurse's comment, which for some reason caused me to wonder what others will be saying about me. What blessing could there be in having two cancers and now two surgeries within a month, with one being a fluke? How do I say I trust God and so much is happening one after the other? I could not have avoided this intestinal surgery nor having a rare type of breast cancer. I felt like I was losing ground in the hope department as the thought of my dashed hope for my brother's healing came back to haunt me.

As I sank deeper in doubt, I found myself asking the questions, "Am I being punished for something? Lord, what am I missing? What do you want of me?" After days of soul searching, one day in the midst of my praying on the issue, I heard the words, "Have you considered my servant Job?" whispered in my heart. If you wonder who Job is – you can find an account of his life in a book with the same name in the Bible. The question that I heard can be found in Job 1:8 and again in Job 2:3.

"And the Lord said of Satan, "Have you considered my servant Job, that there is none like him on the earth, a blameless and upright man, who fears God and turns away from evil?" Job 1:8 KJV

Although God thought very highly of Job, Satan was given permission to attack him. The first chapter of Job's book documented Satan's attack on Job's possessions and his children. In the second chapter, he attacked Job's health – and there was where I stopped and meditated. I found comfort as I was reminded that I am in the care of one greater than I can ever imagine. I also found comfort in Job 2:6, "...and the Lord said unto Satan, behold, he is in thine hand; but save his life." (KJV)

The Cure Is In The Living

In all I had been through and currently going through, I was still living. I had a chance to exercise positive thinking; I still had the opportunity to be fearless in the face of trials.

I was discharged two days after surgery, and on the morning of Monday, January 27, 2020, just before 7:00 a.m., I woke up from this dream.

I was in a room with three male and three female doctors. The male doctors were standing together as a group and the same for the female doctors. The Male group was going over my case regarding breast cancer and the thought of removing the whole breast versus removing only the affected areas. The female group, while listening, had an 'I am not really interested' demeanor. I stood up and asked about the belly flap procedure I had learned about when I went for my 2nd opinion. Everyone looked at me as if I broke some rule by speaking, especially the women. The lead male doctor finished talking, and the three women left the room without saying anything. The male doctors remained in the room with me and started to speak with me about the case, so I asked if they think the 2nd opinion that I had received from the female doctor was worth looking at more closely. I mentioned the slide that they had used to demonstrate how it could be done when he asked me, "which slide." So I told him, "the same slides you gave me that I took to the 2nd opinion - you should still have it." The other two doctors gathered around the computer as he tried to pull up the slides on the computer.

I woke up with the realization that the Baptist team had three women, and I had encountered three men from Moffitt, so I figured I got my answer as to which procedure I should do.

Chapter 20—Back On Track

I was ready for my January 31, 2020 office sit-down at Moffitt because I had a level of confidence that I knew what needed to be accomplished. After the usual meet and greet formalities, the doctor went over his recommendations again and asked if I had any questions. I then shared that I had a second opinion and explained to the best of my 'no medical experience' ability how to remove the affected areas without it being a full mastectomy.

He was hesitant at first as he shared concerns for the procedure, with the main one being 'preserving my quality of life.' But because I believed the lumpectomy was best, I kept asking questions. Eventually, he decided to examine the area again.

"Actually, now that I see the area again, I think that could work."

You know what was going through my mind at that point – right? "Why didn't he examine me again before trying to convince me it would not work?" Before we had a final decision on this procedure, he had to consult with the other doctors that would be involved in the process.

I left the office and decided to invite my son Mikey to lunch since I was in the area. Plus, I had good news to share. The restaurant was not as crowded as expected for lunch, so we were seated quickly. As we eased into our seats at the high table for two by the window, Mikey asked me how I was feeling from the abdominal surgery, which was an excellent lead-in to my office visit and the now delayed surgery.

We were still waiting for our order of chicken lettuce wraps and shrimp bowl when the breast surgeon called to say that they agreed that this was the best option for me when viewing my overall situation and especially after all I have been through.

"Thank you, Jesus!" I yelled as the waitress was placing the plates before us.

"I am sorry it took so long," the young lady stated with an odd expression on her face.

"Oh no, that was not because of the wait – I just received some good news," I responded, realizing the reason for her apology.

By now, Mikey was also confused. "We have a plan," I said to him, fast-forwarding to the procedures that were to come. The doctor's notes from that conversation read:

'After reviewing the films with radiology, I have agreed to perform a right central lumpectomy (using a wire to mark the posterior extent of disease), as well as a Savi, guided excision of the positive node. I believe this less extensive surgery is reasonable when reviewing her case as a whole and respects the patient's wishes.'

Placement of the wire and Savi was more traumatic for me than the surgery; at least for the surgery, I was asleep and could feel absolutely nothing. After one of the appointments, I was overwhelmed by what needed to be done and the discomfort of the procedure itself that when I got back to the waiting room, I just sat in a corner and cried uncontrollably.

Before long, it was February 19, 2020. The day of surgery was upon us, and I was present to get prepped for my 'right needle localized central lumpectomy, right Savi Scout localized excision of an axillary node.' My son Mikey, his wife Jen, and Roger occupied the few chairs in the room.

As we waited quietly and patiently for my turn, I tried to figure out the gown I was wearing. It was different from any hospital gown I have ever worn to cover my body.

Chapter 20—Back On Track

It was made of what appear to be two layers of durable paper -like material. It totally wrapped around me, and although it was made of thick paper, it was not rough to the skin. The gown was attached to a portable unit that blew air into it through specialized air channels with tiny perforations. It also had a controller that I could use to adjust the temperature depending on how I felt. It would inflate slightly depending on how high I had the control set that I joked about floating off the bed if I was not careful. Overall, it worked wonders for my menopause inspired temperature fluctuation. So I was good.

I was jerked out of my thoughts by a snickering sound coming from Mikey's direction. "Well, mom, if hospitals were giving frequent flyer miles, you would have a few free surgeries by now." I can always depend on this child to look at the financial aspects of things.

Eventually, it was my turn. The doctor came in, met the family, and reassured me everything would be fine, and there would be no change to the procedure before he disappeared around the corner. Next, my surgical team made the same introductions. They let me know what they would do, and then off I went to surgery—been there done that, right?

It took a bit longer than expected for me to wake up from the anesthesia this time. The nurse called me a cheap date. All that was important was that I was alive. The surgery went well. I was awake and on my way home by mid-afternoon. I was bandaged and secure in my after surgery pink support bra, along with a prescription for Hydrocodone to handle the pain.

Previously it was determined that the cancer was triple-negative, and my doctor told me chemotherapy was my only choice. When I insisted I did not want chemotherapy, he appeased me by saying we can cross that bridge when we get there, but first things first, performing the surgery. Well, surgery was over, the pathology report was they got all cancer out and tested lymph nodules were clean. But I was now at that preverbal bridge and needed to decide if I take the recommended preventative treatment.

My appointment on March 6, 2020, was to determine what treatment was best for me. The doctor for my consultation was very nice and friendly. He referred to me as a 'lovely 60-year-old female', but I think he changed his mind when I would not give in to the recommended chemotherapy treatment.

Since the treatment for the lung cancer that had metastasized is working and the newly diagnosed breast cancer was surgically removed (although noted that it is aggressive), I chose not to get chemotherapy but will take every test available to catch it early if it ever returns.

Chapter 21

The Choices We Make

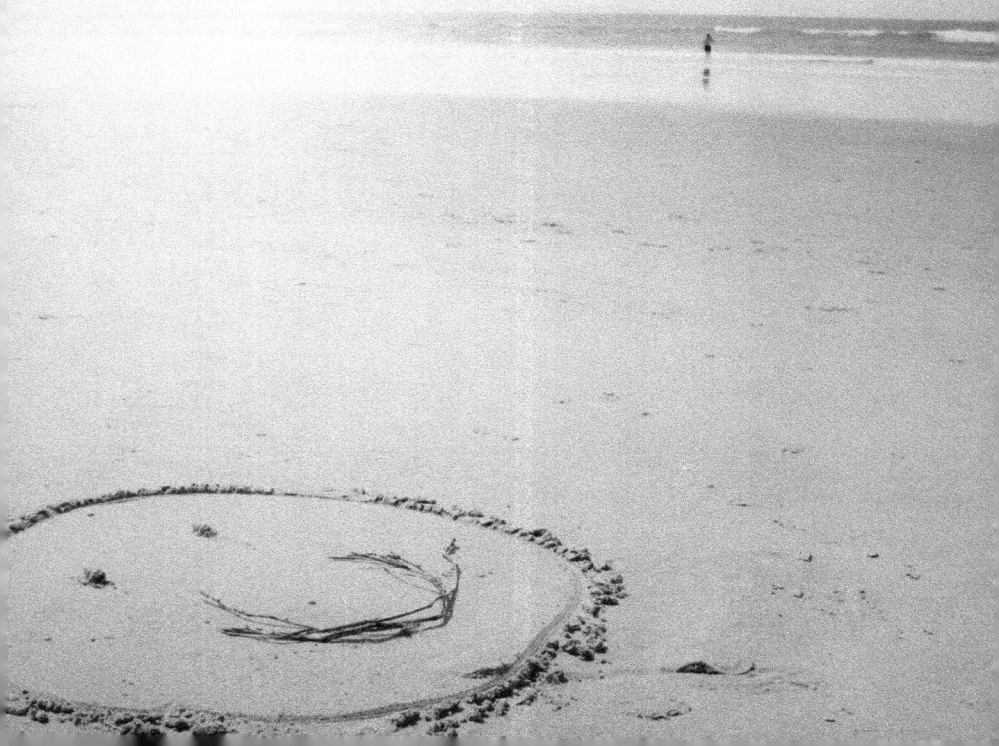

In the past, I would work for a goal and get to the place where I hoped to be, then find out that I had lost because the goal was no longer an option. On this journey with cancer, it would appear that I had lost from the first day I received my diagnosis, but here I am, realizing that I had gained.

I learned the meaning of living instead of merely existing. The first thing the Lord revealed to me was that I invest too much mind space into what others think about me. The amount of time I had spent trying to be liked by those I allowed in my life was draining the very thing from my body. Instead of satisfactorily fueling me, it was killing me.

I had to accept that everybody's fight is not mine, especially while they fold their hands and watch with no pretense to fight for themselves. I can remember when I succumbed to my friend's plea for me to help her find job possibilities. She was out of a job, so I gave up my weekend to search the internet for positions that matched her preferences. I weeded through job listings on multiple websites, which took me into the evening; I was exhausted. I later found out that while I was looking for a job for her, she was partying at a club.

Apart from my multiple surgeries that seemed to take every bit of strength I had to hold on to my hope in Christ, I made it to the year 2020. Once again, I lived to witness new life – the birth of Mikey's daughter – my second grandchild. Due to the pandemic, months passed before I could hold her, but a view from the window and pictures became the acceptable norm.

I can still remember the many media posts referencing the 2020 vision and the clarity that will be obtained for the coming year. For some, I believe they hoped they did have a clearer idea a few years back because this one started with an element of unease.

The Cure Is In The Living

There was the impeachment of the 45th President of our United States. He was charged with abuse of power and obstruction of Congress only to be acquitted by the US Senate.

To me, whether or not he was guilty took second place to my horror of how the members of the US Congress behaved. The representatives who were put in place to protect the people from a government abusing their authority were destroying the very thing they should be defending by the scandalous way they conducted themselves. What can one expect when the jury had already decided the defendant was not guilty before the case was presented.

Before long, I decided to withdraw myself from the news to preserve my sanity. It is amazing how everyday events can trigger or deposit stress in your life. After hearing the arguments and the verbal fighting, I felt that it was not worth the effects it had on my mental health. I had heard enough to know how to pray for my nation; God knew this day would come just as he knew who would hold the political offices. Ironically, I had accepted that there were fewer presidents and politicians for me to see than what I had already seen. Still, my anxiety was for my children and grandchildren; to think of the world that was ahead of them. After all, if the gatekeepers of the law are lawless, then what will the people do? Who will protect them from those who make decisions that determine how they live?

Twenty-twenty (2020) had also ushered in the coronavirus outbreak, which was first identified in Wuhan, China. The coronavirus disease 2019, abbreviated as COVID-19, was new and not previously seen in humans. By December 2020, the death toll in America had surpassed over 300,000 deaths and was rising. It became a pandemic that literally affected all corners of the world, causing churches,

Chapter 21—The Choices We Make

business, school closures, and the cancelation of public events. Job losses and anxiety of parents having to home school their children were at an increase.

Personally, I did not quarrel with the rules. They said to stay home; restrict the number of people gathering together. Wear your masks and exercise social distancing where words you hear every single day without fail. I was considered high risk, so whatever the guidelines, I adhered to them. How silly it would have been that I had fought and survived the numerous health issues over the years just to be brought down by Covid-19 because I disobeyed the guidelines. It was a chance I was not willing to take.

I am sorrowful for those who accused others of having a lack of faith because they refused to go to church during the pandemic. I know my faith was strengthened during that time. I was able to spend more time in prayer and God's word as I sought his guidance. I was blessed abundantly during this season. I missed the birth and the first two months of my second grandchild, but no matter how much I wanted to see and hold her, I respected the social distancing concept.

I always had a place in my belly where I felt the Spirit of God occupied. When it felt empty, I knew I was not as close to him as I should be. When the place felt extremely full, I knew something was coming up that I would have to turn over to him. And there were times when the overwhelming feeling was just because I loved Him. I have a feeling for no one else but God the Father, Son, and Holy Spirit.

At age 60, this was the year when I finally understood the love of my birth mother, Clair. I can count on one hand the number of times I saw her face to face, but we communicated by letters and phone calls sporadically throughout the years. We had a relationship, but I never felt that mother-daughter connection.

The Cure Is In The Living

It happened on an overseas telephone conversation on May 2, 2020, with Clair when I asked her to recall the day she left Jamaica and how she felt that Sunday afternoon. I was careful not to say 'when you left me behind' not wanting to influence the answer. One Mississippi, two Mississippi, three Mississippi the seconds ticked on as I waited patiently for the reply, not wanting to miss even the slightest inflection in her voice. By the time she spoke again, I realized that she paused, not to recall, but to fight back the hurt she still felt 58 years after that day when she left me behind.

This response was another reality check as I wondered how different my life would have been if I had not harbored the misguided feelings I had for her over the years. It was also another incident where God showed me an area in my life that needed forgiveness. I was then able to totally forgive her and feel the release of that burden as I asked the Lord to forgive me for not doing it sooner.

To think all those wasted years of mistrust, misdirected hate, overzealousness of wanting to be liked and needed. Not to mention the constant internal struggle with feeling I do not belong and the hard work in trying to prove that I do belong. Could all those now unsubstantiated issues have contributed to my poor health? Actually, I don't think I have poor health. Apart from cancer cells trying to destroy my body, I considered myself healthy.

I read an article that said stress has a profound impact on how our body's systems function and that it makes your body more hospitable to cancer (Lorenzo Cohen, Ph.D. professor of General Oncology and Behavioral Science)

I found another internet article written by Yasemin Saplakoglu, which stated: 'Past research has also shown that during a stressful situation, the body turns on two key pathways: the sympathetic nervous system, which triggers the

Chapter 21—The Choices We Make

fight or flight response, and the hypothalamic-pituitary-adrenal axis, which releases a key stress hormone called cortisol...Past research has shown that chronic activation of both of these pathways can lead to hypothalamic-pituitary-adrenal metabolism changes, increased levels of certain hormones, and the shortening of telomeres; the caps of the ends of DNA that prevent damage. All of these changes could potentially influence the development and progression of cancer.[1]

Another bit of information I came across was an interview conducted with Dr. J. Clark. He explained the biblical and scientific effects of toxic and negative emotions and the connection to our nerve system. I had a 'wow' moment when she made the statement "the negative emotions of childhood becomes the diseases of adulthood." (Something More program, https//youtube.com/opvduxhu0ha)

Now that I had been afflicted with two different types of cancers, when was the seed planted? Was it that day when I said, "Knowing me, I will get cancer?" Did I speak badly over my life, or was it a prophetic statement - my divine destiny? Could I have done anything different to change the course? If my younger self had not decided to keep her emotions suppressed but channeled them more productively, would I be a different person? I could waste the rest of my life trying to figure that out and not make a difference.

Yet, with all my research and reading on what causes cancer, each time I ask myself the question: "What could I have changed in my life along the way that would have directed a life of great health?" the answer will always be, "I will never know." But, if I ask the question of what I could have done differently to live a happier, fuller life, boy do I have a list. The first item would be to reduce stress, followed by another long sub-list of changes needed to minimize stress before getting to my second item of the main list.

Most of my experiences and emotions, or lack of, allowed me to clearly grasp and feel a real difference with my love for God. At times it makes me feel like dancing and shouting; I get excited talking about his goodness and faithfulness. I don't simply think I cannot live without him; I know I cannot do anything without him.

My prayer time often ends with tears of joy as I feel such an outpouring of love for my Heavenly Father and his love for me. There is no doubt within me that my love for God surpasses every other feeling I have had for anyone or anything. I was set free of thinking I should feel and express myself like others did when I understood the precious gift I had. I did not only know about Christ; it was not just an infatuation; instead, I was totally engulfed in his true love – and I have experienced his grace.

Even so, I wanted to experience more of God's presence in my life and started by personalizing and repeating Paul's prayer in Ephesians 1:17-19 and 3:14-19. But I did it reading from the GNB translation where the words first came alive and clear to me. And so day after day, I repeated (don't forget now, this is my version as I personalized Paul's prayer):

"God of our Lord Jesus Christ, the glorious Father, I pray that you would give me the Spirit, who will make me wise and reveal God to me so that I will know him. I ask that my mind may be opened to see his light so that I will know what the hope to which you have called me is, how rich are the wonderful blessings you promise your people, and how very great is your power at work in me who believe."

Chapter 21—The Choices We Make

Then, I went on to the next set of verses in chapter three and prayed:

"My heavenly Father, from whom every family in heaven and on earth receives its true name, I ask you God from the wealth of your glory to give me power through your Spirit to be strong in my inner self, and I pray that Christ will make his home in my hearts through faith. I pray that I may have my roots and foundation in love, so that together with all God's people, I may have the power to understand how broad and long, how high and deep, is Christ's love."

And because I believed in the revelation from Psalms 118:17 and not being ashamed to proclaim what the Lord has done, I also prayed from Ephesians 6:19-20 (GNB):

"God, I pray that you will give me a message when I am ready to speak, so that I may speak boldly and make known the gospel's secret. For the sake of this gospel, I am an ambassador. Help me to be bold in speaking about the gospel as I should."

I don't know if it was the answer to those prayers, but in March 2020, I found myself in deep prayer during one of my morning devotions. I recall that I was still in my bed with a bible and a few books next to me but not sure what led me to such intense prayer that morning. With tears leaking from my closed eyes suddenly, I had a vision of me standing at the bottom of a hill looking up at an image of Jesus on the cross. The realness of the moment allowed me to feel a level of compassion and a greater appreciation for the sacrifice and God's love than I had ever felt before. My belief that Jesus died on the cross rose from the dead and the fact that He will return someday was strengthened even more.

At the time, I did not know how much I would need to hold on to that extra boost of feeling connected and loved by God.

The Cure Is In The Living

Chapter 22

A Test Like No Other

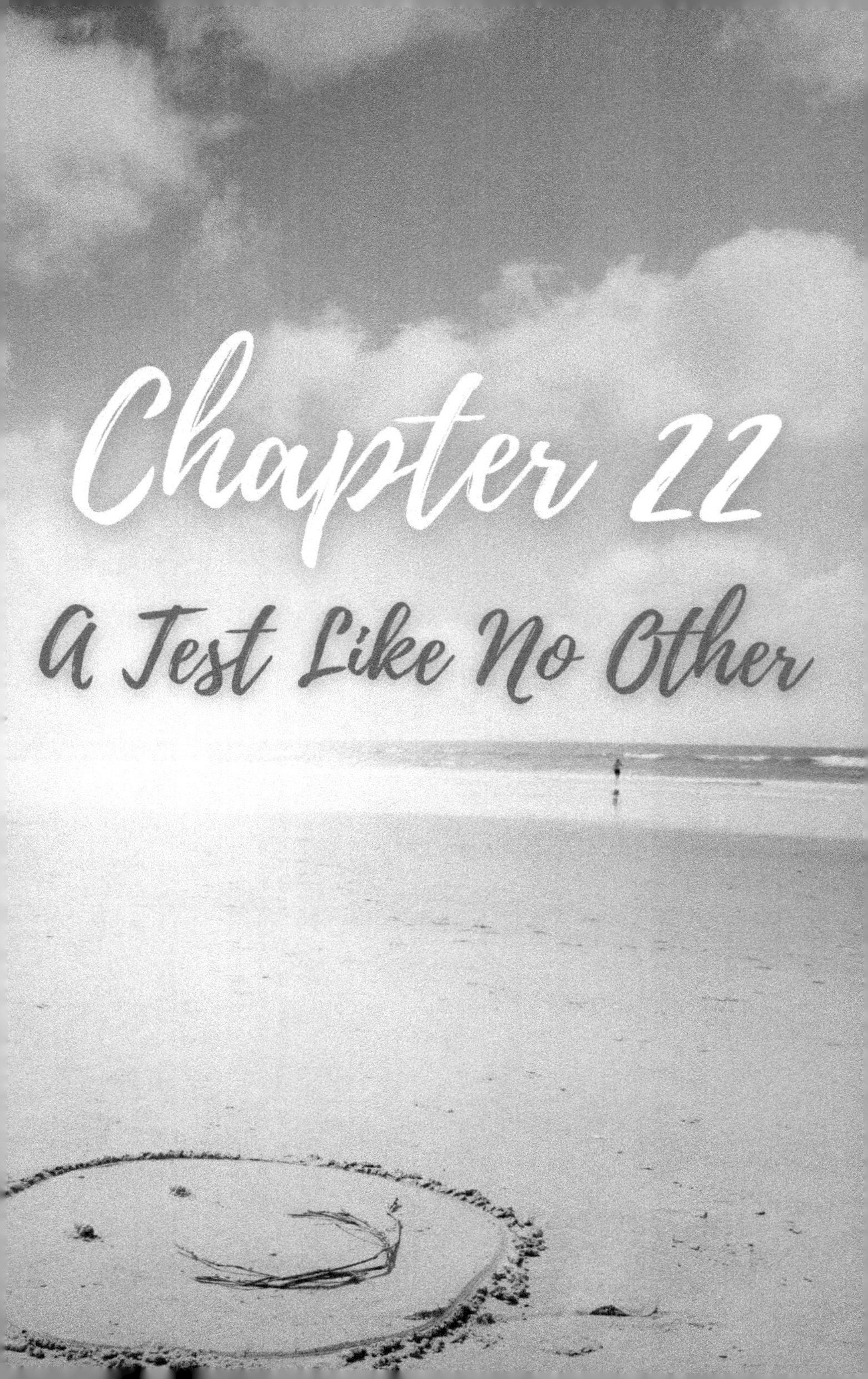

On July 16, 2020, I found myself back under the microscope because it appeared that the breast cancer had resurfaced. Yep – it has been only five months since the previous breast lumpectomy. A few weeks prior, I did my usual self-exam, and I felt a small mass but thought it was scar tissue from surgery. My doctor ordered an MRI just to be safe, and there I was. I am in an all too familiar place – getting a special mammogram for confirmation. To think I went ten years cancer-free, and now I couldn't make it to one year – what is happening to me?

I was alone again when I got the mammogram results. The finding was 'numerous hypoechoic masses within the right central and right lower outer quadrant breast appear suspicious.' I knew the next step – the dreaded painful needle -guided biopsy. I prayed for it to be nothing, but the biopsy results revealed evidence of cancer. After getting the news, I felt hopelessness creeping in as I asked myself the question, "Is this the last leg of the journey? Did I make a mistake by not having the full mastectomy with the first surgery?" Then I remembered that the 2nd opinion was that if I did not have chemotherapy, the cancer would come back sooner than later. I did not have the chemotherapy treatment.

Pity parties were never a part of my makeup, so within a few minutes, I took a few deep breaths. I thought, *If this is the end, I am going to get ready for it.* I walked to my closet and gazed in for a while before going to the garage to get an extra-large heavy-duty garbage bag. When I returned to the closet, I examined every piece of clothing and filled that garbage bag with items I felt would be a blessing to someone else.

Twenty minutes into my task, I got to the end of the first row and paused. The next item was a baby blue lace dress with each laced flower outlined with a white thread piping. With both hands on my hips, I stared at the formal outfit that I had purchased several years ago to be worn to Nathan's wedding. They had decided not to have a formal wedding after all, so the dress was slated as a possibility for Mikey's wedding because he was also engaged. By the time Mikey's wedding came around, they had a semi-formal spring garden wedding, so the formal dress did not make that event either.

As I reached back up and pulled the dress from the rack, the result from a suppressed mixture of fear, anxiety, and hopelessness had reached the base of my throat, and I could feel tear ducts ready to explode. "Well, you missed two weddings; maybe you were waiting for the funeral." I smiled as I put the dress back in its place.

It is indeed devastating to hear the words 'YOU have cancer,' and it has crippled many. In past cancer announcements, I was determined not to allow my mind to go to that place of hopelessness. I knew I had God on my side and never failed to profess my faith in Him over the years. Testimony after testimony left my lips to the ears of anyone who would listen. I told of the miracles I had experienced throughout my life. Why did this news hit me so hard? Where did my 'get up and brush yourself off mentality go? There I was, with all my faith and belief in a sovereign God, and all I could feel was weakness, failure, and loss – my loss.

Thank God he was not through with me yet.

But his answer was: *"My grace is all you need, for my power is greatest when you are weak." I am most happy, then, to be proud of my weaknesses, to feel the protection of Christ's power over me." II Corinthians 12:9 (GNB version)*

Chapter 22—A Test Like None Other

The thing about God's words of comfort is that sometimes it requires us to be in the waiting area for a period longer than we want to be or can understand. I could not join in with the Apostle Paul's response because I was not feeling happy or proud of my weakness but oh how I desperately craved to feel the protection of Christ's power again. I needed it now.

During a conversation with my publisher, he mentioned a documentary on cancer he came across some time ago. My search for the documentary did not provide what I expected, but I found a book with a similar title, so I bought that instead. To my surprise, April, the author, lived in a neighboring county. Both hands and a shout of praise went up to the Lord – I was amazed by my findings. My hope for treatment was being restored.

April wrote of her crazy cancer and the holistic journey she chose, which proved successful for her. My hope was further heightened when I saw her doctor's name, who was also from the same area. I often had read of clinics having a cure, but they were usually far away from my residence, so this was a fantastic find. I did my due diligence on both the doctor and April. By the following day, I had an appointment with the doctor and left a message for the author to call me back – and she did. She was still doing well, six years after she published her book. She was not a celebrity or spokesperson selling a product but was still working at her insurance company. What kept us from meeting in person was that we were at the heights of the Covid-19 pandemic. Nevertheless, I had a real person close by to speak with who had gone through the holistic approach and was doing well.

Dr. John Young of Clearwater, Florida, suggested that I first do the RGCC test, commonly called the "Greek test." They would use my blood to identify circulating tumors and cancer stem cells in my body. The results would provide information about the types of treatments that would work best for me – in accordance with my personal DNA. It provided types of natural supplements and even types of chemotherapy that would work with what was going on in my body.

Dr. Kiluk and I had another heart-to-heart talk at my next visit to discuss the upcoming mastectomy. My request to see pictures of similar surgeries did not pan out very well. What I thought would have helped me prepare for the outcome brought more anxiety, so I asked if I could speak with a Psychologist before the surgery. He wholeheartedly agreed, and it turned out to be one of the best decisions I made. I recognized within myself that I was not ashamed to say I was seeing a Psychologist. Another positive outcome was when I shared my testimony regarding my anxiety and decision to seek professional help. Doing so propelled two others to seek help for personal issues they had been struggling with for many years.

Once again, I learned something about myself. I was spiritual and confident regarding the relationship I had with God, but there came a time when that relationship was tested. Christians often put on a brave face and pretend that all is well when they are suffering inside. It took months for me to forgive myself for being doubtful and so ready to accept the hint of defeat. I was able to do so when I realized that my faith was not shaken during it all. Obviously, even a believer can have times of doubt. And guess what – it is okay as long as we do not faint along the way. As long as it is possible, I will keep the mindset that even if I have one day left, I will live those hours for the glory of God and to the best of my ability.

Chapter 22—A Test Like None Other

Mikey was also thinking along those lines and pitched the idea for a weekend on the beach. He knew how much I loved the ocean, so he and Nathan planned a mini family vacation. It ended up happening just two weeks before my next scheduled surgery. I had the opportunity to spend a long weekend with my sons, their wives, and most of all, my precious granddaughters. To top it off, the house that Mikey found for our getaway was literally a few yards from the beach. Each evening we watched the beautiful sunsets, and at night I sat on the beach listening to the crashing waves, looking at the stars, and praising God for how great He is.

One night, seated in lounge chairs with the ocean before us, and sand-covered feet, Nathan and I held hands as we prayed a prayer of thanksgiving. Another night Mikey and I took a long walk on the beach but on our way back, it started to rain heavily. By the time we got back to the house, we were drenched; but I was so happy to have had the joyful experience of walking in the rain on the beach. I was so thankful for that weekend because both occasions with my sons were additional blessings, which will always help to make the dark days not seem so dark after all.

The reality is with all I have suffered from humans and sicknesses, it has always been about me and not them or the disease. The cure rested securely in me and how I chose to walk it out. It took a very long time for me to realize that, but what a blessing it was when I did.

The text of II Corinthians 12:10 (GNB) brought me to that place:

"I am content with weaknesses, insults, hardships, persecutions, and difficulties for Christ's sake. For when I am weak, then I am strong."

The Cure Is In The Living

Whenever the stench of death surrounded me, I sought and received more strength as I focused on living. A woman once said, after her mother passed she realized, she spent a lot of time trying to get her to appointments and administering her medication and meals that she missed the final days of life with her mother. It is so easy to focus on the disease that we forget to live the time we do have.

The surgical procedure recorded as '...mastectomy... removal of palpable axillary nodes' was completed on October 12, 2020. I was still groggy when Dr. Kiluk came in to tell me that the surgery went well and what to expect for the upcoming days. When he was through talking, I thanked him, reached over and touched the area where my breast once was, and cried my last tear for the loss. It was time to heal and move forward.

The devil has no authority over my life, and I was not about to give it up for free. My mind was on Christ Jesus – I believed with everything I knew and had that he was in control. I sought his face for answers to every question that came up. I decided to fight for every hour that God had for me, and giving up was not an option.

It was not a matter of trying to cheat death; in fact, I had said many times that there would come a day that I would die. Even Lazarus, whom Jesus raised from the dead, had to die eventually. What I wanted to ensure, though, was that I lived a life whereby I was able to fulfill God's purpose for me and not miss the mark due to premature death. And for those who might say there is no such thing as premature death, I say it does not matter. What mattered was my view – what I believed. Ecclesiastes 7:17

I heard a radio announcer say, "If my presence has no value, then my absence won't make a difference." It was a version of Trey Smith's quote. I typed up those words and

Chapter 22—A Test Like None Other

displayed them where I could see them every day. If we do not truly know our value as revealed by God, our creator, we will continue to exist and breathe each day but never truly live.

I have seen others get extremely emotional to the point of tears as I share my testimonies and often wondered why? I don't seem to feel burdened by the things I had endured. At the end of each trial, after a while, I usually find a blessing. Each incident had allowed me to prove God's goodness and miracles, and it was always an overwhelming joy to experience them. Then one day, it hit me as I heard that whisper, "You did not feel the burden because God has been carrying you through."

The fact is during cancer or any illness that we may find ourselves having to endure, the defeat or the joyful prize is not in the disease or the healing but in the living. We should not have to die trying to live. Gaining wisdom, knowledge, and understanding is a part of living; it brings peace to your situation. For me, it was staying in the right spiritual frame of mind, so I would grab every event and safety line the Lord threw my way. I tried to make sure nothing he sent me fell by the wayside. I would prefer for my children to say, "She tried and failed," than to say, "She gave up too soon."

I lived my life before cancer and experienced unpleasant and painful times. And with cancer, I continued to live day by day; whether in tears or laughter, I lived. Cancer became another step in my life's journey. I had my worst and best financial issues during cancer. I had my greatest struggles and joys with my children after I had cancer and painfully watched as they struggled to make it as well. One man left me, and another found and truly loved me when I had cancer.

The Cure Is In The Living

In the final analysis, life's elements did not care that I had cancer, so I lived it. I lived to see Barack Obama, the first African American president who served that office for eight years. I also lived to see the swearing-in of Kamala Harris, the first African American woman (with Jamaican blood to boot) and first female vice president, making her the highest-ranking female official in our Country's history.

I found stability in the words of Philippians 4:12-13: *"I know what it is to be in need and what it is to have more than enough. I have learned this secret so that anywhere, at any time, I am content, whether I am full or hungry, whether I have too much or too little. I have the strength to face all conditions by the power that Christ gives me." (GNB)*

And I will keep striving no matter where I find myself until I no longer have the ability to do so.

Sharing and caring for others is a part of living as well. I found boldness in doing for others as it is placed in my heart to help or support them. In this area, I had to overcome the fear of someone taking advantage of my resources or time. I found confidence in Joseph's words in Gen 50:20 when he told his brothers, "You plotted evil against me, but God turned it into good to preserve the lives of many people who are alive today..." As long as I am able to do good for someone, I will do it without fear of losing. God knows my heart, and if I should misunderstand his directions and am being used, he will turn it around for good.

My goal was to do God's will, not to live in fear. Only He knows all things and the minds of those that present themselves before me. I realize it was in knowing God and trusting Him, even to the point where it may appear stupid, that I had been able to make it this far. Through that unquestionable 'trust,' I realized that I was able to share God's goodness in ways that He was glorified by the life he gave me.

Chapter 22—A Test Like None Other

In hindsight, regardless of the medical procedures, you choose to follow, do not forget to also serve God, your creator, and live the life you have. Be bold, non-judgmental, do not harbor negative feelings, and feel free to laugh at yourself. No one is perfect.

The good I find in my bout with cancer is that I am cognizant that my days are numbered. I might not know that final number, but I am fully aware that the clock is ticking, and it feels like it's ticking faster than usual.

I have no idea when my journey will end, but I am sure I will have God with me all the way. But until that time comes, I choose to look at the rose instead of the thorn; I choose to enjoy the rain as I do the sunshine, I choose to live and bask in God's love and thrive. I will continue to lift hands in praise and thanksgiving to God for keeping me for so many years. I will continue to love and sing and laugh and dance and, in the same manner, continue to forgive others as Christ forgave me. We live in an imperfect world among imperfect people.

I may never forget the beginning of this journey, the tears, what I was doing, where I was standing when it sunk in that cancerous cells were found in my body. My immediate regret had been the possibility of never seeing my four-year-old and my 4-month-old babies grow up. And now I can rejoice because the Lord kept me to see them both married, being great husbands and fathers. I had an opportunity to love on my granddaughters Mya and Olivia. Among all that I have done in my life, raising Mikey and Nathan has been my greatest accomplishment. But to have lived to see them carving their way through life has been a greater blessing.

And so I have no regrets; cancer has not been a curse but has propelled me to higher heights and deeper depths in my relationship with the Lord. I cannot regain the steps I have already made, but I sure can change the one I am about to take. I lived when I could have died. It continues to be an amazing journey, and as of today, February 20, 2021, as I write the last sentence in this book, it is not yet over. The very first time a doctor told me there was evidence of cancer in my body was more than 30 years ago and counting. How marvelously blessed I am to be alive.

The New Beginning...

Scriptures

to Remember

SCRIPTURES REGARDING HEALING

"Lord, by such things people live; and my spirit finds life in them too. You restored me to health and let me live." *Isaiah 38:16 (NIV)*

"Heal me, LORD, and I will be healed; save me and I will be saved, for you are the one I praise." *Jeremiah 17:14 (NIV)*

"But I will restore you to health and heal your wounds, declares the LORD, because you are called an outcast, Zion for whom no one cares." *Jeremiah 30:17 (NIV)*

"Nevertheless, I will bring health and healing to it; I will heal my people and will let them enjoy abundant peace and security." *Jeremiah 33:6 (NIV)*

"Is anyone among you sick? Let them call the elders of the church to pray over them and anoint them with oil in the name of the Lord. And the prayer offered in faith will make the sick person well; the Lord will raise them up. If they have sinned, they will be forgiven. Therefore confess your sins to each other and pray for each other so that you may be healed. The prayer of a righteous person is powerful and effective." *James 5:14-16 (NIV)*

"Praise the LORD, my soul, and forget not all his benefits— who forgives all your sins and heals all your diseases, who redeems your life from the pit and crowns you with love and compassion," *Psalm 103:2-4 (NIV)*

"The LORD sustains them on their sickbed and restores them from their bed of illness." *Psalm 41:3 (NIV)*

"LORD my God, I called to you for help, and you healed me." *Psalm 30:2 (NIV)*

"He heals the brokenhearted and binds up their wounds." *Psalm 147:3 (NIV)*

"Have mercy on me, LORD, for I am faint; heal me, LORD, for my bones are in agony." *Psalm 6:2 (NIV)*

"A cheerful heart is good medicine, but a crushed spirit dries up the bones." *Proverbs 17:22 (NIV)*

"Worship the LORD your God, and his blessing will be on your food and water. I will take away sickness from among you," *Exodus 23:25 (NIV)*

"See now that I myself am he! There is no god besides me. I put to death and I bring to life, I have wounded and I will heal, and no one can deliver out of my hand." *Deuteronomy 32:29 (NIV)*

"My son, pay attention to what I say; turn your ear to my words.   Do not let them out of your sight, keep them

within your heart; for they are life to those who find them and health to one's whole body." *Proverbs 4:20-22 (NIV)*

GOD FORGIVES US

"For God so loved the world that he gave his one and only Son, that whoever believes in him shall not perish but have eternal life. For God did not send his Son into the world to condemn the world, but to save the world through him. Whoever believes in him is not condemned, but whoever does not believe stands condemned already because they have not believed in the name of God's one and only Son." *John 3:16-18 (NIV)*

"Let the wicked forsake their ways and the unrighteous their thoughts. Let them turn to the LORD, and he will have mercy on them, and to our God, for he will freely pardon." *Isaiah 55:7 (NIV)*

"God made him who had no sin to be sin for us, so that in him we might become the righteousness of God." *2 Corinthians 5:21 (NIV)*

"In him we have redemption through his blood, the forgiveness of sins, in accordance with the riches of God's grace." *Ephesians 1:7 (NIV)*

"You were taught, with regard to your former way of life, to put off your old self, which is being corrupted by its deceitful desires; to be made new in the attitude of your minds; and to put on the new self, created to be like God in true righteousness and holiness." *Ephesians 4:22-24 (NIV)*

"If we confess our sins, he is faithful and just and will forgive us our sins and purify us from all unrighteousness."

1 John 1:9 (NIV)

WE MUST FORGIVE OTHER

"For if you forgive other people when they sin against you, your heavenly Father will also forgive you. 15 But if you do not forgive others their sins, your Father will not forgive your sins." Matthew 6:14-15 (NIV)

"But to you who are listening I say: Love your enemies, do good to those who hate you." Luke 6:27 (NIV)

"Do not judge, and you will not be judged. Do not condemn, and you will not be condemned. Forgive, and you will be forgiven." Luke 6:37 (NIV)

"Bear with each other and forgive one another if any of you has a grievance against someone. Forgive as the Lord forgave you." Colossians 3:13 (NIV)

"Hatred stirs up conflict, but love covers over all wrongs." Proverbs 10:12 (NIV)

"For though the righteous fall seven times, they rise again, but the wicked stumble when calamity strikes." Proverbs 24:16 (NIV)

"And when you stand praying, if you hold anything against anyone, forgive them, so that your Father in heaven may forgive you your sins." Mark 11:25 (NIV)

Thank you for reading! Always remember,
The Cure Is In The Living!

Visit **TheCureIsInTheLiving.com** for more info

www.ingramcontent.com/pod-product-compliance
Lightning Source LLC
Chambersburg PA
CBHW020607270326
41927CB00005B/214